Funeral Service Exam
SECRETS

Study Guide
Your Key to Exam Success

Funeral Service Test Review for the
Funeral Service National Board Exam

Published by
Mometrix Test Preparation
Funeral Service Exam Secrets Test Prep Team

Written and edited by the Funeral Service Exam Secrets Test Prep Staff

Printed in the United States of America

This paper meets the requirements of ANSI/NISO Z39.48-1992 (Permanence of Paper).

Mometrix offers volume discount pricing to institutions. For more information or a price quote, please contact our sales department at sales@mometrix.com or 888-248-1219.

Mometrix Media LLC is not affiliated with or endorsed by any official testing organization. All organizational and test names are trademarks of their respective owners.

ISBN 13: 978-1-60971-768-1
ISBN 10: 1-60971-768-6

Dear Future Exam Success Story:

Congratulations on your purchase of our study guide. Our goal in writing our study guide was to cover the content on the test, as well as provide insight into typical test taking mistakes and how to overcome them.

Standardized tests are a key component of being successful, which only increases the importance of doing well in the high-pressure high-stakes environment of test day. How well you do on this test will have a significant impact on your future- and we have the research and practical advice to help you execute on test day.

The product you're reading now is designed to exploit weaknesses in the test itself, and help you avoid the most common errors test takers frequently make.

How to use this study guide

We don't want to waste your time. Our study guide is fast-paced and fluff-free. We suggest going through it a number of times, as repetition is an important part of learning new information and concepts.

First, read through the study guide completely to get a feel for the content and organization. Read the general success strategies first, and then proceed to the content sections. Each tip has been carefully selected for its effectiveness.

Second, read through the study guide again, and take notes in the margins and highlight those sections where you may have a particular weakness.

Finally, bring the manual with you on test day and study it before the exam begins.

Your success is our success

We would be delighted to hear about your success. Send us an email and tell us your story. Thanks for your business and we wish you continued success-

Sincerely,

Mometrix Test Preparation Team

Need more help? Check out our flashcards at:
http://MometrixFlashcards.com/Funeral

TABLE OF CONTENTS

Top 20 Test Taking Tips

1. Carefully follow all the test registration procedures
2. Know the test directions, duration, topics, question types, how many questions
3. Setup a flexible study schedule at least 3-4 weeks before test day
4. Study during the time of day you are most alert, relaxed, and stress free
5. Maximize your learning style; visual learner use visual study aids, auditory learner use auditory study aids
6. Focus on your weakest knowledge base
7. Find a study partner to review with and help clarify questions
8. Practice, practice, practice
9. Get a good night's sleep; don't try to cram the night before the test
10. Eat a well balanced meal
11. Know the exact physical location of the testing site; drive the route to the site prior to test day
12. Bring a set of ear plugs; the testing center could be noisy
13. Wear comfortable, loose fitting, layered clothing to the testing center; prepare for it to be either cold or hot during the test
14. Bring at least 2 current forms of ID to the testing center
15. Arrive to the test early; be prepared to wait and be patient
16. Eliminate the obviously wrong answer choices, then guess the first remaining choice
17. Pace yourself; don't rush, but keep working and move on if you get stuck
18. Maintain a positive attitude even if the test is going poorly
19. Keep your first answer unless you are positive it is wrong
20. Check your work, don't make a careless mistake

Sociology/History

Visitation

The social and religious rituals are separated into three categories. The first ritual has to do with the practice of visitations. Family and friends gather to visit the body of the deceased. The casket can either be open or closed. Often this practice is linked to the condition of the body or the wishes of the family members. The visitation is scheduled a day or two prior to the funeral service. In the following days the funeral will be scheduled. Attendees are given the opportunity to pass by the casket for the purpose of viewing during open casket ceremonies. The funeral service officiator, pastor, or priest may lead the congregation in prayer. Eulogies, Bible readings and hymns may also be an important part of the funeral service. The burial will take place after the funeral ceremony.

Burial practices

The body is moved to the cemetery or place of burial. When the body is buried in a cemetery the final act of the funeral service takes place at the cemetery. There are several options for those that wish to be buried. The body can be placed in the ground or in a tomb or crypt. Those that have served in the armed forces may be buried in certain location of the cemetery reserved for the military. Members of the Armed Forces honor their dead with a draped flag over the casket, the playing of the taps on the bugle, and with a gun salute. The draped flag is given to a spouse or parent before the casket is lowered into the ground. This is followed by the playing of the taps and the firing of the rifles to honor the military service of the deceased.

Types of service

A **eulogy** is a reflection given to honor the deceased discussing fond memories and accomplishments achieved by the person during their lifetime. Members of the Catholic or Anglican faith do not allow the giving of the eulogy in their services. **Adaptive** is a service that veers away from the traditional rituals. The service is changed to reflect either the person's religious or social customs in some way. A **humanistic** service veers away from all religious conventions or ceremonies. **Neo-traditional** services veer away from the more traditional or long standing approaches. **Memorial services** are given when the corpse is not available for the ceremony. Instead, the attendees will view photos of the deceased. Mementos and music is usually associated with this service. Deceased persons who have served in the military may also have the military honored rituals performed during this service.

Funeral Rule law

The Federal Trade Commission protects the consumer in the selection of the services that best fits his or her personal requirements. The role of the funeral director during this time is to inform the consumer about the goods and the services along with a price list. The price list must be given to the consumer in a written or verbal format. Consumers must be given this list before seeing the product. Individual pieces may be purchased. The products may also be packed in a "package deal". However, the consumer has the option of purchasing either individual pieces or the package.

This right must also be written on the price list to ensure that the consumer is aware of this practice. Certain items are required by state and/or local law and must be clearly marked on the price list forms.

Consumers have the right to purchase caskets from other dealers. If that is the case, the funeral director does not have the right to refuse the use of that casket. The funeral director may not even charge a service fee for the handling of the casket purchased elsewhere. In addition, whenever there is cremation services provided there must also be alternative container options. Alternative containers are inexpensive containers that are made from either wood, pressed board, or fibrous materials. The cremation service allows the body to be disposed of through fire and extreme temperatures. This method turns all the organic material found in the body into ashes leaving only the bones to be processed. The bones go through a grinding process. The remains are then placed into a box to be given to the family and friends.

Impact of industrial world

Before the advent of the Industrial Period in history, families consisted of a more patriarchal nature. Fathers held the leadership role within the family. The nuclear family was the most common family type at that time. Mothers worked within the home as homemaker and as the caretaker of the family. Women were expected to care for the husband and children, to cook, and to clean. In many instances, fathers were present or close at hand throughout the day. This allowed the father the opportunity to fulfill a role of leadership within the family unit. However, the Industrial Period changed the family structure as the father left the home to work in factories and in other positions that became available. The father's absence from the home positioned the mother into a more authoritative role of leadership in the family unit. The once patriarchal family structure changed to a matriarchal family structure.

Must behaviors

Must behaviors are patterns of behavior that are followed at the onset of a death of a person within a society or family unit. There are three types of must behaviors that regulate the person's conduct in times of grief. The three types of must behaviors are **taboos, mores,** and **laws.** Laws are governmental enforcements of a rule. The breaking of laws can result in punishments to be served by the offender. Taboos are not as confining in that there is not governmental enforcement if a taboo is broken. Still, these do restrict or prohibit certain behaviors in regards to the customary rituals regarding death. Mores consist of the principled ideas that call for a certain action and treatment of the deceased in accordance with societal beliefs. The adherence to these "must behaviors" are usually held in accordance with the person's belief system and the law of the land in which they reside.

Family authority figures

The matriarchal authority describes those family units that are run by the mother. The mother's role has increased in leadership since the advent of the Industrial Age. The onset of the World Wars further advanced this role of leadership. Fathers were away across the ocean. Mothers were left as the single authority in the home during that time period. The father's role of absolute authority declined as a result of these rather difficult circumstances. When the fathers returned to the home after the war, many of the women found they were not satisfied to return to their old roles within the home. The Patriarchal unit where the father was the absolute authority was no longer as popular. In some instances, a more Egalitarian unit developed. Mother and father shared in the parenting roles with equality. This gave the family a financial boost when women entered the workforce.

Ethnocentrism and cultural relativism

The funeral director should be equipped to provide grief counseling and facilitate funerals for a wide variety of people. The funeral director should understand that ethnocentrism is marked by an emotional response based on a person's customs, attributes, or language base. Divisions among people are marked by the belief that their own race or culture is superior to others. In cultural relativism the belief is held that all cultures deserve to be treated with equality. These differences can be critical in helping a funeral director meet the needs of the family and friends of the deceased. The director must remain impartial and treat the consumers with fairness regardless of any personal biases. The funeral director may be called upon to provide counseling services that do not offend a person's ethnological beliefs.

Folkways are the everyday behaviors that are considered the norm by society members. Folkways are not strictly enforced. However, some of the aspects of violation of a folkway involve ridicule, criticism, and reprimands. The habit of sending a sympathy card is one example of a folkway. Another example is in the bringing of prepared food after a death. Many cultures allow for this folkway to be practiced. The food is prepared and brought to the home of the family of the deceased. This folkway allows the friends and family that have prepared the food to express their sympathy to the family of the deceased. Dressing in a specific color can be considered a folkway in some cultures. Years past, widows were required to wear black for an extensive period of time. Failure to do so resulted in recriminations.

In the **Jewish society** the *Taharah* is a ceremonial ritual that is performed to prepare the dead person's body for the coming rituals. The Jewish communities have their own burial societies which are responsible for the *Taharah*. The burial society is known as the *Chevra Kadisha*. The *Chevra Kadisha* begins with a prayer of forgiveness for the deceased. This is followed by total immersion of the body into a warm bath. The head is washed first. Then the right side of the body is washed. This is followed by the washing of the left side of the body. Finally the back is washed. The body is dried and dressed in a white linen outfit. The adorned body is placed into a pine box. The heart and genitals of the deceased are sprinkled with dirt that originated from Israel, the Jewish homeland.

Diplomacy

A funeral director must have the skills of a diplomat and maintain a role of impartiality, especially when parties are not of like mind. The funeral director should listen to the feelings and ideas presented by each family member. Then the director will summarize the conversations of all parties leaving off the point of contention. This point of contention will be given consideration through a diplomatic discussion of the significance of the options. Each option will be discussed in detail. The terminology will be explained to ensure that all parties understand the meaning of each service and product. The director strives for an amiable agreement between the parties. However, the person(s) that are responsible for the financial aspects of the funeral are the ones given the ultimate choice in making the decision. In some instances, a judge may have to make the final decision.

Reactions to grief

Many people experience anger in response to the loss of a loved one. This anger may be directed at the loved one that has died. The grieving person may feel frustration, abandonment, or resentment. Occasionally, this anger is directed at other family members. The grieving person may hold the opinion that others are not exhibiting the proper response to the death of the loved one. Some even blame the death of a loved one on an attending physician or other responsible party. Yet another emotion that is often experienced is one of guilt. Guilt is the result of the unresolved issues that the deceased person and the grieving person did not have the opportunity to settle. Guilt may be the result of a misperception by the survivor that the death could have been averted by some action on his or her part.

Many people experience powerlessness and hopelessness over the death of a loved one. Some exhibit signs of sleeplessness, disrupted sleep patterns, or an overpowering sense of loss. Still others can become extreme violent and moody. Others become overly sensitive. Persons that are overly sensitive may withdraw socially during this time. Others may experience withdrawal and become extremely depressed. It is not uncommon for people to experience lethargy. Some have periods of troubling doubts, even going so far as to question their faith and belief systems. There are some that become incapable of expressing their emotions during this time. The funeral director must take into consideration all of these factors in dealing with the family member who exhibits these reactions to their grief. The director should remain diplomatic and sympathetic during their encounters with the grieving family members.

Denial is a normal reaction when a person dies suddenly or violently. Denial begins as a coping system for the person that is grieving. The mind shies away from the shocking thought of the loss and begins to deny the reality of the loved one's death. Denial is the first step in the grieving process. The person in denial is experiencing a type of shock. This coping mechanism may even allow the person an appearance of calm and control. However, it is important to realize that this may only be the initial stage of the loss. This period of denial can be of short or long duration. Many religious and cultural groups can be of an enormous comfort to the person experiencing a loss. Viewing the body may reduce the length of time that the grieving person experiences denial.

The grieving process is one in which an emotional release must be reached by the loved ones of the deceased. Writing the death announcement can have a high psychological benefit to the grieving party. The funeral rite allows those who are grieving to express their sorrow over the departure of their loved one. The idea that the deceased person is resting peacefully is comforting to the grieving person. This idea is enhanced when the grieving individual has the opportunity to view the body. Sometimes circumstances will not permit the viewing of the body. In these cases it is beneficial to make the funeral arrangements. This helps the person to accept the death and escalates the grieving process. In accepting the death of the loved one in this manner, the person can finally deal with the death and bring closure to the event.

Cremation

Cremation can be traced to approximately 3000 B.C. This was the period of the Stone Age. Cremation rituals were elaborate and ornamental in nature in the Slavic countries. The Slavic rituals gave credence to the practice and over time the ritual spread to other countries. Trade migrations in the Bronze Age increased the acceptance and introduced this practice to other parts of the world. Britain and Spain began to accept this ritual into their death ceremonies. The Mycenaean Age of 1000 B.C. gave rise to the practice in Greece. This ceremonial death ritual was well accepted due its expedient nature of dealing with the deceased body. Romans further spread this practice into parts of Italy, Europe, and Asia. Constantine Christianized the Empire and denounced the ritual as a pagan ritual. Thus, burials were more widely practiced over the course of the next 1500 years.

Death and dying

The study of death and dying from a psychological and sociological viewpoint can be examined through the thanatological viewpoint. Every culture remains constant in their treatment of honoring and respecting the dead. In the United States, we have a multitude of cultures with different belief systems. Social, ethnic, economic, and religious factors can be reflected in the way that a person or group deals with a death. For instance, some African American cultures may conduct a ritual ceremony that honors the dead with singing, drumming, and a procession as the dead body is transported to its final resting place. The ceremony is directly linked to the cultures belief concerning their dead ancestors. The importance of this ritual as well as many other rituals for other cultures is the act brings closure to the surviving relatives and friends.

Social structures

Social structures within a family can be constructed from a basis of beliefs regarding religion, law, class, or economics. Other factors can be related to the family's social structure as well. Families can be described as single parent families, nuclear families, extended families, the family of origin, or the family of procreations. Mothers can hold the leadership roles. Fathers can also hold these roles. Other leadership roles are split as in the Egalitarian model of a family. This concept of a family's social structure is ever-changing in our modern world. The position as funeral service director is one in which diplomacy should be paramount. The successful director will be able to recognize and adapt to the needs of a wide variety of cultures. The director should maintain an attitude of honor and respect to the deceased and the survivors of the deceased.

History

The **Roman funeral** began with the expectation of the demise of the decease. This caused the happenstance of the next of kin to sit beside the dying person. The person present at the time of death would cover the mouth of the decease to catch the dying person's last breath. Then the deceased person's eyes were closed. A coin would be placed over the deceased person's mouth to honor *Charon*, the ferryman of Hades. The deceased was settled onto a sofa of ivory and gold for nine days with his feet facing the door. The funeral service was held at night. Musicians would play music and sing. Actors would emulate the deceased. Freed slaves would attend the funeral wearing the hat of the deceased. Images of the deceased, crowns, and military awards were displayed. The practice of cremating the body became more accepted in latter years.

Embalming was part of the **Ancient Egyptian's** religious belief system. The embalming served a practical use as well. The Nile River was known for its flooding tendencies. The embalming provided a sanitized method of dealing with the corpse. The first method required that the brain be removed from the head cavity. Then the head would be packed with resin. Evisceration is a term to describe the removal of the internal organs. The resin washed organs would either be placed into canopic jars or into the body. The body would be packed or immersed into natron or sodium salt. Immersion would last for a period of 20 to 70 days. The fourth step required that the body become dehydrated. The dehydration process took place under the extreme temperatures of the sun. Finally, the body would be wrapped into a mummified state.

Formaldehyde use

F. D. Blum discovered a substance that produced a hardening effect in 1893. The substance that produced this effect was called, "formaldehyde". This substance could also be used to disinfect and to preserve. Dr. Auguste Renouard published, "*The Undertaker*" in 1878 where he discussed the substance. The first permanent school was founded to promote the use of embalming and the products used in the process. This was known as the United States College of Embalming. Dr. Auguste Renouard was the demonstrator for this school. However, he did purchase the school at a later date. The Rochester School of Embalming marked the modern age of embalming. However, it should be noted that formaldehyde is not to be used without caution. Formaldehyde has a pungent odor and can lead to serious health risks. Risks can include serious breathing problems, headaches, and other ailments.

Cooling boards

Cooling boards were used from the 1880's on up until around the 1940's. The cooling board was a board on which the body was laid. Underneath the cooling board would be a slab of ice. This slab of ice allowed the body to stay cool until burial. Some cooling boards had holes drilled on the top to allow the ice to reach the body. Others had tops that consisted of a cane material which allowed more of the cool air from the ice to penetrate to the body. Still others had a covering over the top which served to enclose the body within the cool air. One manufacturer of this board was B. F. Gleason. Boards without holes were more than likely to have originated from those who used the cooling boards in their homes as part of their embalming techniques.

Fisk Metallic Burial Casket

Originally coffins consisted of a wood material. Cabinet makers in the 18th and 19th century often found work available as coffin makers whenever cabinet making was not in demand. James A. Gray was the first to obtain a patent for his coffin made from a metallic substance. Almond D. Fisk's metallic burial casket became more popular than Gray's. Fisk placed a window in his casket that allowed the survivors to view the deceased. The glass window was positioned at the head of the casket. The metallic casket had the ability to be sealed and then was filled with a preservation liquid to prevent decaying. This gave families the opportunity to transport deceased members over longer distances. It also assisted in cases where normal embalming methods were not advisable as in the cases of death by mutilation, etc. Henry Clay and Daniel Webster highly endorsed this product.

Important People

Frederick Ruysch: Frederick Ruysch was born in 1638. As a Dutch anatomist, his specialty was in the preservation of body organs. He published his findings and included dioramas displaying the composition of body parts within the skeletal framework. His work was unusual in that he would create botanical landscapes made up from the body parts. Worms would be recreated from intestines. Trees or shrubbery would be represented by the use of veins. He discovered a dye that would allow persons to view the pathway of blood in the organs. He would use the decorated tops of baby jars to display animal specimens. His work or curiosities dealt with the brevity and complexity of life. His images were displayed along with music, candlelight, and refreshments. This atmosphere was used to elaborately show off his exhibits. His work was also known as the 8th Wonder of the World. He died in 1731.

Anthony von Leeuwenhoek: Anthony von Leeuwenhoek was a tradesman. However, he made fantastic discoveries with the use of a microscope. He discovered bacteria, protists, sperm cells, blood cells, nematodes, and rotifers. These microscopic discoveries were revealed with the use of the microscope. He furthered his discoveries by learning how to grind and perfect the microscope's lenses. He further advanced the field of microscopic research by developing over 500 microscopes with a wide range of capabilities. One of his advancements allowed the magnification of 200 times. His descriptions are remarkably detailed concerning these specimens. His descriptions include illustrations. His findings were illustrated by a contractor that he employed. The drawings hold the distinction of being instantly recognizable as the various specimens that he discovered. Anthony von Leeuwenhoek was a remarkable man that furthered the field of research for the scientific community.

Edwin Chadwick: Edwin Chadwick's work established sanitation procedures necessary in the fight against epidemic diseases. The White chapel authorities of London, England enlisted Edwin Chadwick's help in the fight against the epidemics of the time. In 1842 Chadwick published a report on the subject of sanitation. The first Sanitation Commission was appointed due to Chadwick's self-published work. A textbook on sanitation and reform was created out of this event. His findings directly linked the advent of epidemic diseases to the degree of unsanitary conditions that people were subjected. His findings concluded that poverty held a huge impact upon the ability of persons to provide proper drainage, cleansing efforts, and proper ventilation of the living environments. Persons more affluent could more readily afford to sanitize and remove the noxious agents from their living space. His findings indicated that removal of unsanitary conditions did produce a reduction or eradication of diseases.

Jean Gannal: Jean Gannal was a French chemist who wrote "Histoire des Embaumements." Dr. Richard Harlan worked as a translator to produce an English version of the "Histoire des Embaumements." Jean Gannal's book became the first book published in English and distributed in the U.S. on the subject of embalming. The book stirred up a huge controversy over the use of arsenic. Arsenic is a poisonous substance that was used as one of the ingredients in the embalming fluid. This fluid could pose a serious threat to the students that dissected the embalmed cadavers. Gannal did not retain the patent rights to the method of insertion of embalming fluids into the body. His highly publicized court case concerning the carotid arterial insertion of the fluid proved that Gannal was not the one to first come up with this method of insertion. Gannal did obtain a patent in 1847 for an embalming solution.

Dr. Thomas Holmes: Dr. Thomas Holmes worked as an embalmer during the Civil War. His experiments earned him the title as the" Father of Embalming". He used a chemical solution for embalming over 4028 casualties of the Civil War. President Lincoln promoted his work in an effort to return the dead soldiers to their homes for burial. Dr. Holmes offered this service at a rate of $7.00 for the enlisted men and $13.00 for the officers. His work was in such a demand that he resigned his commission to begin his work as a civilian. He found it necessary to hire salesmen to solicit the families of the north and the south to purchase coupons. The coupons would be carried by the soldiers into battle. Dr. Holmes and his assistants would search the dead bodies for the coupons. His advancements in arterial preservation increased the practice of embalming the dead.

Important Institutions

<u>International Conference of Funeral Service Examining Boards:</u> The International Conference of Funeral Service Examining Boards is responsible for the procedures and licensing of Funeral Service Administrators. This agency began in 1903. The discussion of transporting dead bodies across state lines became an issue that had to be dealt with by a multitude of state authorities. State licensing boards gathered to discuss how best to transport the bodies across state lines. In 1928 the accreditation of mortuary schools was considered. By 1930 the accreditation of mortuary schools along with state licensing procedures was established. The exam covered examination needs, death care information, and funeral service education. The agency provides a direct certification process, presentations, seminars, and a national convention. This agency holds the funeral industry personnel to a set of high standards in an effort to promote a standard of integrity for the profession.

<u>ABFSE:</u> The American Board of Funeral Service Education (ABFSE) is an organization that is responsible for funeral service educational programs. Originally, the ABFSE was entitled The Joint Committee on Mortuary Education. The ABFSE has held the sole responsibility of providing certification to its members since 1962. The Board works to provide educational opportunities that meet the standards of the funeral service education. Likewise, the Board's accreditation is tied to this objective. Furthermore, the accreditations of related fields are obtained from this board. This accreditation is necessary to those who wish to work in the field of the funeral industry as this is the only acceptable accreditation available. These hard earned accreditations are recognized by the Funeral Director's Association and by the International Conference of Funeral Service Examination Board.

Important terms

Blended Family: The joining together of both mother and father with their children from previous marriages along with the children from the existing marriage.

Casket: The preferred terminology in reference to a coffin or box used for the burial of a body.

Cemetery Plot: A small section of ground in which the casket will be buried.

Cemetery Property: The sections of cemetery plots, crypts, or columbaria that are used to house the deceased remains.

Cemetery Services: The services provided that allow for the maintenance required in a cemetery. Some services provided include: the opening and closing of graves, crypts, and/or niches; setting markers, grave liners, and vaults; lawn care services; and the maintenance of structures found on the property.

Class: The terminology used to refer to the social and cultural status of a group.

Columbarium: A set of niches that are used to house the cremated remains of the deceased.

Contemporary: Persons that live in the here and now or the present time period.

Crypt: A building or structure found above ground on the cemetery property that can hold either a single body within a tomb or a series of bodies in multiple tombs. It is not uncommon to find a family tomb which houses the deceased members of a family.

Cultural Relativism: This term implies that all cultures deserve to be treated with equality.

Culture: The word used to describe the social belief system of a group of people of shared customs and ideas that can have a direct or indirect impact upon that group.

Customs: The word used to describe the social behaviors that are associated in a traditional way within a particular society of people.

Demographic: The information that is provided in statistical form regarding the number of births, deaths, marriages, income levels, and other data in relation to a certain population.

Disposition: This is the act of placing the deceased remains (either a body or the cremated remains) in the final resting place or destination.

Egalitarian: The sharing of equal authority by male and females in regards to one's duty and leadership.

Extended Family: The mother, the father, their children, the wives and children of the son's within the family. This does not include the married daughters' husbands or children.

Family of Origin: Your birth family.

Family of Procreation: a family unit that is produced by having children with your spouse.

Folkways: The common practices of a particular society in their everyday life.

Funeral Rite: The terminology used to describe all the formal and ritualistic activities involved in order to accomplish the funeral.

Funeralization: The method that involves all the details and processes that must be accomplished to perform the final disposition of the body.

Immediate Disposition: The direct burial or interment of the remains without making a concession for any type of ceremony or ritual.

Law: A governmental enforcement of a rule that allows for a punishment to be served if not followed.

Matriarchal: a family unit that places the mother in the role of leadership.

Modern: A term used to describe choices that tend to be current and popular with the times that we are currently living.

Mores: A principled idea that calls for a certain action and treatment of the deceased in accordance with societal beliefs.

Nuclear Family: The portion of the family unit that consists of the father, the mother, and their children.

Patriarchal: A family unit that places the father in the role of leadership.

Religion: A belief system that functions within a set of behaviors, customs, and/or rituals.

Rites of Passage: The term given to important ceremonies that symbolizes events such as marriages, baptisms, or funerals.

Ritual: a ceremony that allows the participants to express their emotional and behavioral responses to a death of another person.

Rules: Policies or stipulations that govern the practices or methods used by an organization or group.

Single Parent Family: The children and one parent that make up a family unit.

Subculture: A small group of people with particularly unique traits that are not shared by the larger group in which they exist.

Symbol: An icon that is connected in some way to form a meaningful representation in recognition of a religion, culture, or society.

Taboos: A restriction or prohibition on the performance of certain behaviors in regards to customary rituals.

Psychology

Acute grief

Acute grief can be linked to emotional, physical, behavioral, and cognitive factors. Some people experience grief from losing a job, ending a relationship, losing a pet, or over the loss of their possessions. Research points out that many people experience grief in alignment with their own personality. Many factors trigger grief responses in a person. Family's can have a direct impact on how a person deals with grief. A person's culture or religious beliefs may also influence how a person deals with grief. Bereavement is said to be a natural part of life. A live person can expect that at some point death will occur resulting in the end of the natural life cycle. Extended family relationships, children, marriages, and mental health can be negatively impacted during the mourning process. It is important that a person in mourning seek emotional support.

Stages of grief

Initially it was believed that grief could be categorized into the following stages: **denial, anger, bargaining, depression**, and **acceptance**. However, research has evolved to include processes and dynamics. One such addition is construed out of a need for self-preservation. The shock or numbness or sense of unreality may even appear as strength. The next process includes a yearning and searching for the person that has been lost. It is not unusual for a person to search the crowds for the face of a lost loved one. This yearning is also known as "pining away" for the loved one. Disorganization and despair is another process of grief. This is recognized as depression, and mourning of this type can last for years. The culmination of this process ends with acceptance. Reorganization involves the rebuilding of the survivor's life without the presence of the deceased.

Grief process risks

The grief process can be an extremely vulnerable process for a person to go through. Some people experience nightmares during this time. Others experience a loss or increase in their appetites. Still others experience sleep disorders. Some people exhibit repetitive motions that are an attempt to avoid the pain of loss. It is expected that a person may even experience events from time to time that may trigger an emotional response to the loss. Some have been known to have hallucinatory experiences. Their hallucinations usually involve seeing or hearing the loved one come into the room or standing at the doorway in some familiar way. These experiences can be auditory, visual, olfactory, positional or gustatory in nature. These sensations may be evident a year or two after the event. If these sensations continue or worsen after a lengthy period of time, a person should seek professional help.

Types of bereavement

The major types of bereavement that are most common include: **childhood bereavement, death of a child**, and the **death of a spouse.** Children that range in age from 8- 12 months old may experience a lasting effect from the lost of a parent. This is the age in which children bond closely with their parental figures. Sometimes children are bombarded with confusion as to the permanency of the death. The children may be under the misguided presumption that the deceased parent can be fixed with a medication, a treatment or even that the parent is just away on a trip. Children may also behave immaturely during this time. Some express anger or withdraw. Older children may respond with anger or with repetitive motions such as those found in using computer games. This helps them to avoid dealing with their intense emotions of grief. Some children respond with a physical or mental illness.

Children can die as a result of a still birth, Sudden Infant Death Syndrome (SIDS), illness, or accidental deaths. Many parents never accept the child's death and experience extreme guilt. Often marital problems can result in the intensity of the grief that the parents undergo. Some marriages break up because of the child's death. In more drastic cases a parent may even attempt suicide. Another form of bereavement is caused by the death of a spouse. The surviving spouse often expresses a sense of loss of themselves. The survivor may have additional obligations placed upon them due to the absence of their deceased spouse. Others may find that social occasions are difficult. Some may isolate themselves from social events. Still others are left out of previous social activities involving couples. Many allow that this can be one of life's most traumatic events when the Dyad (two units) has been separated.

Types of grief

Anomic grief is difficult for the survivor because the survivor has not established an acceptable method to deal with the grief. One example of this type of grief can be found when a parent loses a child. The parent expected the child to outlive the parent and has not established a method to deal with the mourning process. The parent can expect to be disoriented over the event. **Anticipatory grief** is expected at the end of a long illness. Death comes as a relief and expectation that life is limited. **Delayed grief** is feelings of loss are put off until the person can cope with his or her feelings at a time in the future. **Exaggerated grief** is a response that causes the person to become motionless or to come to a halt. This is an extreme form of grief. **Masked grief** is exhibited by the person in an unaware state. The person does not recognize that the actions or behaviors being exhibited are a result of the grief being expressed in some way. **Complicated grief** is a type of grief that is chronic and unresolved for a seemingly endless period of time.

Director as facilitator

The funeral service director works closely with the bereaved to help them feel at ease during the process of planning the funeral. The director may offer alternatives or suggestions to help the survivors to adjust to the new circumstances which they are facing. This is not a counseling session. Instead, a funeral service director offers detailed examples and choices for the bereaved family to make. The best funeral service directors illustrate with ease. The funeral service director clearly outlines and explains the products and services being offered. The director does not take an active part in the bereaved decision-making process. This requires a smooth, professional demeanor that is unobtrusive and oftentimes, unnoticeable by the survivors. The client must be allowed to make their own decisions given the available information that is expertly provided by the funeral service director.

Counseling

Grief counseling is used to refer to the therapy sessions that are given to the persons involved in the grief process. The positive results of this therapy allow people to gain a healthy perspective on the circumstances of their loss and to accept that loss in terms of a natural grieving process.

At-Need counseling refers to the funeral director's counseling session regarding the arrangements and products to be used regarding the recent death. **Pre-need counseling** refers to advanced planning of the funeral services done before death in an effort to avoid increased costs. **Client-centered counseling** is when the client takes an active part in resolving his or her part of the problem after seeking assistance with some kind of dilemma. Carl Rogers coined the phrase "client-centered." The counselor must be able to see the client in a realistic way. The counselor must also see how the client views himself. These two viewpoints allow the counselor to gain congruence over the situation at hand. In this way the person is affirmed as an individual and encouraged to grow and strengthen healthy attitudes. **Crisis counseling** is therapy that addresses a short-lived or temporary need of a person that is unable to function because of the intensity of grief being experienced. This grief may be displayed in terms of confusion, pain, or other strong emotions. **Directive counseling** is therapy that is given by the counselor in the form of questions and by a suggestion of a possible solution to the problem that gives the counselee a set action to take. **Informational counseling** is therapy in which the counselor shares knowledge pertaining to the problems or subjects that are of a concern to the individual or group being counseled. **Situational Counseling** is a therapy that expands upon Informational Counseling through the exploration of feelings that are tied to certain events or circumstances.

Webster, Jackson, Rogers, and Ohlsen

Webster believed that counseling should be conducted after data from case histories had been collected. His method for conducting a personal interview was varied. He tested his clients for interests and aptitudes. His advice was given as professional guidance after a thorough perusal of the psychological methods in which he applied. Jackson believed that all acts of assistance through a particular dilemma could be considered as counseling that person. Likewise, Rogers' definition of counseling indicated that the communication in which the person involved himself in was of therapeutic merit. Ohlsen made the distinction that those who needed psychotherapy were not those who received counseling. Only those persons who were basically sound of mind could gain benefit from counseling. A person that receives this counseling is said to be the counselee. The person giving the counseling or guidance is the counselor.

Attachment Theory

John Bowlby observed a mother's instinctive reaction in protection of her young during his work. He further extrapolated that the infant's desire to explore and develop was strengthened out of the attachment that the infants had formed for their mothers. This was contrary to Freud's views on the breaking of the attachments formed. Fraley and Shaver went on to say that romantic relationships are in fact relationships that hold similarities to that of infant and mother relationships or attachments. Basically, this theory holds that the desire to experience safety and security is made evident whenever the person in whom an attachment has been made is near. The positive points of the attachment theory are found in the way that a romantic partnership is shared throughout a person's lifetime. However, when the spouse dies, the attachment theory explains that the sense of loss is amplified by this same attachment to the person.

Cognition versus communication

Cognitive ability allows humans the skills to assimilate information and to process that information into a useable form. People use these skills in comprehension, in making deductions, decision-making, and planning. A person's cognitive ability helps them to learn about a variety of concepts. These concepts could include ideas construed within a person's belief system, knowledge, desires, or intentions. These ideas are then communicated in some fashion to others. Communication allows humans the ability to express themselves. People may transfer their thoughts concerning information they have learned. The content or the message of the communicated thought is transmitted to others in many forms. Some forms of communication can include diaries, newspapers, body language, or in some cases, smoke signals. They may also communicate their thoughts through feelings or other actions. The destination of the message is carried out when the intended audience receives the communication.

Unconditional positive regard

The term unconditional positive regard was used by Carl Rogers in his development of client centered therapy. This therapy is based upon decisions made by the client in regards to his or her therapy. The therapist should perform their duties with unconditional acceptance of the client and the problem. The therapist must remain positive and provide encouragement to the client throughout the therapy. The regard that the therapist has for the client is in relation to the client's importance as an individual. The regard includes an atmosphere in which the client can share without fear of condemnation or judgment by the therapist. This atmosphere allows the client to receive the unconditional positive regard that is foundational in giving the client the confidence to resolve his own problems. The client centered counseling session is a non-directive counseling and non-judgmental type of counseling.

Grief therapy

Worden describes the components involved in grief as emotions, physical sensations, cognitions, and as behaviors exhibited. He goes on to describe the problematic issues that are involved in the grief process. Persons that avoid or bottle up their grief are in danger of succumbing to these more complicated forms of grief. Worden advises that the person work towards the completion of four tasks to overcome their grief. The person should work towards accepting that the loss is a part of their reality. Likewise, the person should work through the painful emotions that are a part of their grieving process. The person should work towards making the adjustments to life without the loved one. Finally, the person should work towards an emotional separation from the decease so that the person can go on with their everyday living. The person that works through these four tasks will have completed their grief therapy.

Therapy versus counseling

Grief therapy is reserved for those who are experiencing forms of abnormal grief. Delayed grief, inhibited grief, and prolonged grief are some forms of abnormal grief. The aim of the methods used to assist people experiencing abnormal grief is to help the person to overcome their defenses which are impeding and blocking their natural process of mourning. Grief counseling is a form of reassurance that the survivors are experiencing normal reactions in the grief process. Grief counseling is reserved for the uncomplicated forms of grief. Dr. Alan Wolfelt deemed that grief counseling was a companion for the survivors. According to Dr. Ken Dokathis reassurance is critical to grief counseling. Bereavement caregivers are there to help people cope with their losses and to help them identify the feelings that they are having in the reaction to events or emotions.

Grief Syndrome and grief work

Lindemann describes Grief Syndrome as a normal response to loss. His study was comprised of young survivors who had survived a traumatic fire at the night club Coconut Grove. He believed that the symptoms displayed were ones which shared commonalities among the survivors. Most of those studied experienced the following symptoms: shortness of breath, tightness in the throat, various pains, and a measure of irritability, anger, and lethargy. His study indicated that the grieving process was one in which psychological and somatic responses would be displayed. He further indicated that the survivors would need to work through their grief in order to accept the reality of the loss. Lindemann believed that person in the throes of Grief Syndrome have a very real need to share their feelings in order to accomplish the "grief work" that is necessary for them to become ready to reinvest in life.

Euthanasia

Euthanasia is a Greek word that means "good death". Proponents of euthanasia support the right for people to select the time and circumstances surrounding their own death. There is much controversy over this subject. The term has gained much publicity in recent years. Proponents are usually families of the terminally ill. The terminally ill person selects a relatively painless end to their life that must be administered by another person. This practice is not legal in the United States, nor is it legal in most countries. However, in the Netherlands this practice can be legally performed. In addition, the term "do not resuscitate" or a DNR order is not considered the same thing. This term refers to the withholding of food, water, or breathing apparatus that may prolong the person's life. The DNR order is used when a person has requested that the natural process of dying be allowed.

There are five types of euthanasia. The first type is **direct euthanasia**. The patient is too ill to lift the medication that will end their own life. Another person must directly dispense the medication to the patient. The second type involves an **indirect method**. This occurs when a medical staff provides the drug that can effectively end life. The third type is known as **voluntary euthanasia**. The patient has expressed a desire to take the drug that will end the patient's life. The patient is mentally responsible and fully capable of making their own decisions. The next type of euthanasia is known as **non-voluntary euthanasia**. The patient is fully aware, but doesn't understand that death is imminent. The final type is called **involuntary euthanasia**. The patient or guardian of the person is not in agreement with the action that brings death.

Hospice care

The meaning to the word hospice can be traced back to medieval times. In those days the word was used to describe a place for worn out travelers to find a short respite from the difficult journey ahead of them. However, this word has changed dramatically over time. The word is used to describe the care that the terminally ill receive in the comfort of their home. A team of doctors, nurses, therapists, home health aides, and volunteers service the person that is ill. This service allows the person to stay in the home for a much longer period of time than would normally have happen given the person's condition of poor health. The patient is given the opportunity to stay with their families and to have a more comfortable existence than would normally be given in an institutionalized setting. The psychological benefits of this arrangement are a positive one for the patient.

Nonverbal communication

Nonverbal communication consists of the ability to communicate or share ideas without the use of a verbal or spoken communication process. One person expresses an idea to another person or group of people through the use of body language, facial expression, or through other nonverbal communication methods. The messages may be given in an unintentional or intentional manner. The ideas can be expressed through silence, time expended, proximity, or through the mode of dress. The messages to be interpreted are not always precise. Therefore, the careful application of the commonalities present in the communication must be considered. These considerations should be weighed along with the person's psychological pathways. A person's paralanguage may also be a factor in the communication given. Paralanguage examples can be found in a person's stance, appearance, tone of voice, or pauses within their speech. Nonverbal communication can either substantiate or discredit the verbal communication being expressed.

Thanatology

Thanatology is the study of death and the grief process which the survivors must undergo. The study is conclusive in that it begins with the care that a person receives in the terminally ill stage. This stage is important to the study in that the process of dying can cause suffering to the individual and the family. Death is seen as an inevitable occurrence ending in the final rite of passage. The final dispensation of the body of the deceased is a part of the Thanatological study. The study includes the problems that are caused by the individual's death and how the survivors deal with the loss of the individual. The process of death is viewed from every aspect from the academic viewpoint, holistic beliefs (including positions within the study of humanities), the psychological perspective, the social scientific standpoints, and the cultural perspectives. Thanatophobia is the fear of death.

Needs during loss

Persons who are with a dying person in their last stages of life may experience some relief when they have the opportunity to bid the dying person farewell. According to Worden there doesn't appear to be a purpose in saying goodbye to a person that has already died. Instead, the grieving person benefits more from being able to express their emotions in a quiet room away from distractions. The grieving individual may wish to share their thoughts and emotions. The grief work is a process that must be gone through to help the person adjust to the death of the loved one. Denial and disbelief must be worked through to help the person accept that the loss is permanent and real. The survivor has a real need to withdraw emotionally from the deceased and to reinvest that energy into another relationship.

Humanistic Therapy

Humanistic therapy is a client-directed therapy that is based on the client's ability to find the answers for themselves. This therapy requires the therapist to be a good listener and to be able to paraphrase the statements made by the client. The therapist must respect the client's ability to direct their own therapy. Carl Rogers based his theory upon belief that the approach should allow the person to move towards a healing and growing process that was directed by the client. The client could explore the answers to their problems in a way that fit the client's needs. This process was termed by Rogers as the "predictable process". The counselor recognizes the problem. The client takes control and responsibility for the problem. This allows the client the freedom to discuss the problem and to set his or her own limits. The counselor does not ask questions or provide an opinion.

Conditioned responses

The conditioned response is a learned behavior. Pavlov's dog salivating at the sound of a bell is a prime example a conditioned response. The brain stores knowledge and beliefs, sensory memories and concepts as memories which stem from cause and effect. The consequences to a specific stimulus produce a conditioned response. In the event of a death, the funeral home becomes the specific stimulus which spurs on the memories of another death. This stimulus creates the conditioned response of unease and discomfort or anxiety associated with the death of an individual. There are many such stimuli that can trigger a conditioned response in the case of the funeral rites. One trigger can be in the smell of the flowers which is a sensory memory. Another trigger can be in the singing of a hymn which can relate back to the stored knowledge and belief system of the grieving person.

Causes of grief

Grief and the intensity of grief can be caused by a multitude of factors. The relationship to the deceased may be a factor in the intensity levels of the grief experienced. The level of attachment to the deceased may have long lasting impacts, as well as the relationship with that person at the time of death. Furthermore, conflicts may be a point of sorrow. People may experience anger during this time period. The circumstances surrounding the death may cause feelings of guilt that add to the intensity level of the grief. Sometimes the grieving person's own personality may cause undue stress and raise the level of grief. Certain social situations can add to the intensity level that the bereaved person is undergoing. Other external or internal factors which place stress upon the grieving person may raise the level of grief intensity. These factors must all be viewed as potential problems associated with the grief process.

Bereavement, grief, and mourning

The death of a person is a form of loss which has been defined as bereavement. Bereavement causes the person to be assaulted by a range of emotions. These emotions have been categorized as grief. The grief process has been determined to consist of four classes according t Worden. These are masked, exaggerated, chronic, and delayed grief. Mourning is categorized by a person who experiences grief and is undergoing the process of incorporating the loss into their reality of life. A wife may exhibit her mourning for her husband by reorganizing her life to compensate for the absence of her husband. Worden explained grief syndrome as the condition in which a grieving person produces psychological and somatic symptoms. A person exhibiting a masked grief may not recognize that the actions or behaviors being exhibited are a result of grief being expressed in some way. The most extreme form of grief is found in exaggerated grief.

Affect of grief

The term affect is used in psychological terminology to express an emotional impression within the mind. Affect is expressed outwardly by a person's tone, mood or feelings. In psychology, emotion and affect are often used interchangeably. The range of affect has a range that can be expressed with the use of a monotone voice and no facial expression or through more expressive tones and facial expressions. Affect is unsuitable when it is in conflict with a person's speech or thought patterns. A person may demonstrate mood swings when there are repeated and abrupt shifts of affective patterns. Crying is an outward response to sadness. Sadness is an affect or emotion which is common in the grief process. Other affects that may be exhibited outwardly are feelings of anger or hopelessness. The person may or may not feel comfortable with outward demonstrations of these affects or emotions.

Blame

Blame has three directions or forms in which it can take. The first form of blame is directed at a person or object in an outward or external form. People may direct anger to the cause of the dilemma in an attempt to deflect the blame outwardly. The second form of blame is directed upon the person inwardly. This inward direction of blame is referred to as guilt. Guilt is an affective state of conflict that usually involves a circumstance surrounding the deceased. Forgiveness can be the solution to the guilt process. However, many have a difficult time coming to this realization as the death has prevented the person from seeking the forgiveness from the deceased person that is necessary to curtail the guilt. The final direction of blame is directed at the person who is the receiver of the blame. This form is called shame.

Lindemann's Grief Syndrome

The physical symptoms of grief have been proven to be common qualities in those who suffer from grief. Lindemann reported these commonalities in his outline of 1944. The first form of symptoms includes forms of somatic distress. Somatic distress may come in waves or at intermittent times lasting from a period of twenty minutes to an hour. These symptoms include tightness in the throat, a choking reaction, or a shortness of breath, sighing heavily or often, a feeling of emptiness in the stomach region, a lack of muscular power and vitality, an intensive pain or tension in parts of the body. These physical conditions are a real and a valid complaint among those who suffer from Grief Syndrome. The grieving individual may not even be aware or only vaguely aware that they are exhibiting signs of somatic distress associated with Grief Syndrome.

Tasks of Mourning

The Tasks of Mourning were discussed in detail in Worden's book published in 1991, *Grief Counseling and Grief Therapy*. There are four tasks involved in the mourning process. The first task is in the acceptance of the event. It is not uncommon for the bereaved to spend time searching for the deceased in an effort to try to understand the finality of the death and the loss of that person. In the second task, the person is trying to deal with their everyday life. However, there is a physical and emotional pain that is a part of their everyday existence. The person is trying to stay busy in order to keep from thinking about the loss. This is a task that can be very difficult as the person tries to cope with their everyday life compounded with the stress of pain and loss.

In the third task, the person is adjusting to the environment in which the deceased person is not a part. The survivor must perform the tasks previously accomplished by the deceased. This can create anxiety over the new responsibilities while at the same time cause the person to feel a buildup of frustration and anger that the person is no longer with them to do the work.

In the final and fourth task, the survivor must emotionally break off the ties to the deceased. This break allows the survivor to get on with their own life and to form new relationships with people. This can be difficult when loyalties to the decease cause the survivor to feel as if they are betraying the deceased in some manner. The person feels as if they have dishonored their loved one that has died.

Stages of dying

Elisabeth Kubler-Ross developed the stages of death and dying through her studies surrounding the dying process. She saw a pattern emerge in her studies. She believed that these stages could be applied on a universal level with room for variations for each individual. The first stage involves the stage of denial and isolation. A person may isolate themselves from the situation. One example of this is when a person does not visit the death bed of a loved one out of avoidance of the situation. Many people avoid situations in which they are unsure of how to react or to respond. The next stage is one of anger. In some instances, a person may be angry with God for letting a situation occur. In other instances, the person may be angry at the environment, doctors, nurses, or friends and family members.

The person may feel that no one else is going through what they are going through with quite the same intensity. The next stage involves the bargaining stage. This is the stage in which the person is usually having an internal argument with God. The person is trying to make a bargain with God over their impending death. The next stage involves depression. A person in this stage expresses regrets over past losses. Reactive depression is expressed in terms of lost jobs, lost hobbies or a loss of mobility. Preparatory depression is expressed in terms of future losses that are expected. Preparatory depression is expressed in terms of a loss of independence resulting in a more dependent posture upon the family members. The final stage is one of acceptance. This form of acceptance is one in which the person has come to terms with the inevitability of his or her own death.

Children and grief

Grief in children can be expressed in a variety of ways. Age can be an important factor in this expression. In 1996 Phillip Rice determined the three stages that a child undergoes when a parent dies. The first stage is demonstrated by shock. The next stage is demonstrated as a physical and/or emotional disturbance. This is called the "great disturbance". The third stage is demonstrated by a gradual reawakening. In babies up to age two, there is a sense of loss which may be transferred from the caregiver to the infant. The infant may change eating, toilet, or sleeping habits. Children from two to six years of age may not even understand the concepts of death or time. The child is susceptible to failing to mourn, may personify the death, or have other nonverbal communication disturbances.

Some young children may try to personify death. The personification of death at this age occurs when a person believes that the dead should eat, drink, and perform other natural functions. Some feel as if the parent can come back if the child just wishes hard enough for it to happen. Children from the age of 6 to 9 years old personify death with thoughts of a monster that has taken the parent away. The child may question the causes of death. From ages 9 to 12 years old, the child believes that death is a punishment. The child may feel that previous arguments with a parent caused the death. The child may be apprehension over the funeral, the burial, and have concerns about who will take over the role of caregiver in the child's life.

Suicide

Suicide is the action of ending one's own life. This action has different connotations and a wide range of historical significance. In Japan, suicide was deemed as an honorable solution to a shameful circumstance. Persons have also been known to end their own life as a sacrificial gesture in an effort to save others from some harmful situation. Many cultures see suicide as an act of cowardice and disgrace. The morality of suicide can be argued that the act is one of a permanent nature. However, many of the problems are of a most temporary nature. Not everyone succeeds in their attempt at suicide. Those that fail are known to have made a suicidal gesture. Still others think about committing the act with suicidal ideations. This act carries with it mental health issues and is common only to the human race. No other species ends its own life.

Anomic and Egotistic states

Anomic is the term used to describe how a person separates himself from society. The person in this state can be referred to as a "loner". The 19th Century, French Sociologist, Durkheim first made mention of the term anomic in his book, *Suicide* in 1897. The person that falls to this station has usually come to the realization that he is not in a position in which he can gain an advantage in society. These advantages may be in the form of economical, religious, or societal advantages. The person may end his life or commit anomic suicide because of his feelings concerning his failure to achieve this advantage. The Egotistic can exhibit extreme forms of individualism. Persons without a social contact or social foundational support may commit egotistic suicide because he feels that there is no reason for his existence in life.

Viewpoints

The viewpoints that are closely associated with suicide are the altruistic viewpoint and the fatalistic viewpoint. A person that has a fatalistic viewpoint feels that everything has a predetermined quality. Nothing can be done to stop an event from occurring. The person may seek to commit suicide as a way out of a circumstance in which he or she does not see a resolution. The person with an altruistic viewpoint has a compassion and love for other people. However, the person does not have this same regard for themselves. The person chooses to do well without thought of selfish gain. Some suicides may be a result of the person's desire to bring attention to a bad circumstance. Ghandi's hunger strike is an example of this. A soldier may end his life to save other lives in an act of war. This is known as a Hero Suicide.

Important terms

Acquired Immune Deficiency Syndrome: The transference of a fluid found in blood or semen can aggravate this condition. The HIV virus attack the person's immune system thus causing the problems associated with this disease. The immune system is incapable of fighting off the virus which can cause the infected person to experience symptoms. Illness and infections become the symptomatic problems that the person must guard against. This syndrome can also be passed down from mother to child. A cure for this disease has not been found. However, there are some treatments that have been successful in the treatment process.

Adaptation: The capacity to adjust one's emotional and physiological responses when a beloved person dies.

Affect: The emotional responses experienced and the demonstration of those feelings or emotions.

Aggression: The capacity to act in a hostile or violent manner without provocation. Harm can be expressed in an emotional or physical manner. Some feelings of this type are not carried out, but are simply entertained in the thoughts of an individual.

Alarm: The sudden, and oftentimes, inexplicable feeling of imminent danger or threat.

Alienation: this condition is exemplified by a feeling of isolation or separation. This feeling can be associated with feelings of a lack hope or control over a situation or an event.

Ambiguous Response: Communication in which the receiver is unsure of the meaning. This leaves the receiver guessing as to the intent.

Anxiety: The onset of a negative emotion that involves feelings of panic, uneasiness, fretting, rapid heartbeats, shortness of breath, weakness in the extremities, or a feeling of faintness. The thought pattern in the brain can trigger an emergency response that elevates these sensations in an adverse way.

Articulation: Precise pronunciation of all the sound parts of a word.

Attending: How a person pays attention to their surroundings.

Climate: Emotional tone of how well a message is sent and received.

Concise: Communication in which the receiver is sure of the meaning because the message is clear and right to the point.

Connotation: Emotions brought on by a word or phrase.

Consensus: Group agreement that denotes a resolution to a problem.

Crisis: An event which causes a group or an individual to undergo a period of extreme pain, confusion, and anxiety.

Death anxiety: Describes the person that is undergoing an extreme form of apprehension which causes feelings of deep anxiety and fear to surface in regard to death or subjects that are relevant to death.

Defensive Listening: Technique that involves a person taking offense at innocent remarks to the point in which the person hearing the remarks believes that they are being personally attacked in a verbal manner.

Denial: A form of self-preservation that involves a mental block of the reality of the death or events that are related to the death. The person holds tightly to what is comfortable and "normal" in an effort to avoid the facts that threaten their mental peace of mind.

Denotation: How the bottom line or the end result of the communication is given without any emotional basis.

Displaced aggression: When a person directs the anger over the loss towards a different person or object. This may be a reaction given when the loved one has died. The anger is directed at someone or something present in the moment.

Displacement: When a person directs passionate emotions towards an individual that has no direct responsibility for the situation that has caused the emotional response.

Emotions: The feelings that are expressed by some action or attitude of a person. These feelings can describe the mental state in which a person finds himself.

Empathetic Listening: Technique that involves the assistance of the listener in resolving a problem or crisis that the speaker is experiencing.

Empathy: Having the ability of feeling the same emotion as the other person. This is usually experienced because at some point in your own life you had a circumstance similar to this person's current circumstance.

Environment: Location and history of communication.

Equivocal: Vague, unclear meanings.

Evaluative Listening: Technique that involves a review of the exactness or the useful value of the remarks stated.

Extemporaneous Speech: Casual presentation of material without the use of notes or prepared materials.

Faulty Assumption: Mistaken notion that a message or communication has been given before. This can also refer to the mistaken notion that the message is too hard or simple to comprehend.

Fear: Emotional response that is in anticipation of either pain or danger. This response is usually shown outwardly through an exhibition of dread, alarm, or apprehension.

Feedback: Response given that gives the receiver's reaction to the message that was received previously.

Focusing: Psychological tool used by the counselor to help a person redirect thoughts onto the problem in an effort to the resolution to the problem.

Formal: A speech that has been memorized from a written manuscript.

Frustration: Emotional response that stems from anger whenever a person has lost control of a situation or a goal has not been met.

Funeral service psychology: The study of human behaviors in relation to the funeral services.

Genuineness: How a person expresses heartfelt feelings of a sincere nature.

Grief: A deep and painful feeling of intense loss.

Guidance: Describes how the survivor is taken care of and directed during those times in which solutions to problems must be resolved and decided upon.

Guilt: The feeling that a person has when they feel that the loss could have been prevented in some manner.

Impromptu: A speech that is given without thought or pre-planning or from a previously written script.

Informational Listening: Technique that involves a clear understanding of the thought being expressed by the individual.

Interpersonal Communication: Act of expressing yourself verbally or nonverbally with others.

Intrapersonal Communication: Act of providing a way of expressing yourself independent from others. One form of intrapersonal communication can be found in the use of a diary or journal.

Kinesics: The study of movement or actions that apply to the body gestures and postures that people make.

Manuscript: Word by word deliverance of a prepared speech.

Memorized: A speech that is memorized and given without the assistance of notes.

Message overload: Tons of information that is given which creates confusion concerning the intended message being sent.

Message: Communication given that allows a thought or the action of an individual to be expressed to another individual or a group of people.

Mitigation: The obstruction of an object or a person which is the cause of slowing down the grief process.

Motivation: The mental or physical gratification gained that explains why people act and/or react to circumstances in a certain way.

Mourning: The time period involving the grief process which a person must undergo to arrive at a place in which they can adjust to the loss of a loved one.

Noise: Loud interference that can impede the message that is being sent or received.

Option: The choices given by a counselor to a counselee or client which involves the resolution of the problem being discussed.

Panic: The debilitating feeling that one associates with an intense fear.

Paraphrasing: Restating words to indicate what a person has said without using the exact verbiage of the person.

Pitch: Soprano or bass tones which determine the quality of the speech.

Positive Regard: Acceptance of people as they are without bias or feelings of superiority.

Prejudice: The bias attitudes of a person that rejects the worthwhile attributes of a group, race, gender, or religion and focuses and directs negative experiences on the subject as a whole rather than as an individual.

Projection: The way a person may attribute the undesirable traits or thoughts of another upon someone else.

Proxemics: The study of space and how people make use of that space.

Pseudo Listening: Technique that involves a pretense of attending to the statements made by another person.

Psychiatrist: The medical doctor who is responsible for the treatment and diagnosis of mental disorders.

Psychology: The study of behavior in human beings.

Psychotherapy: Treatments given by psychiatrists or psychologists as an intervention for a person's suffering from mental problems. The professional delves into deeper levels of consciousness with psychological methods that are intended to cure and to improve the person's health. The patient that seeks this treatment on a willing basis is called a client. The person retains the legal right of a patient and must be treated according to the law. Family members may be helpful in discovering solutions to these problems.

Public Communication: A speech given by a person with a small amount of group feedback.

Rapport: The harmony and the accord that can take place in the interactions between people.

Rate: Speed in which the words are spoken.

Rationalization: How people respond in justifying a behavior instead of applying the bona fide reasons behind a particular thought or behavior.

Receiver: The person that is given a message in a communication.

Regression: A coping mechanism in which a person falls into a more familiar pattern of behavior in their management of a particular circumstance or situation.

Relative Terms: The words and phrases that gain meaning from their association or context.

Repression: How a person pushes away or pushes down the conscience thoughts that bring pain to the individual.

Resistance: A coping mechanism in which a person does not try to control either themselves or others in particular circumstances.

Respect: An expression of high regard in which you allow that others have rights as a person of value.

Restitution: How a person will bring about a form of inner equilibrium in which the person finds a way to cope with the reality of the loss in terms of their past, their present, and their future. This is in relation to the theories presented by Simos.

Searching: The thought process which focuses upon the deceased person.

Self-concept: The way a person sees themselves.

Self-disclosure: How a person reveals certain facts Acquired Immune Deficiency Syndrome: The transference of a fluid found in blood or semen can aggravate this condition. The HIV virus attack the person's immune system thus causing the problems associated with this disease. The immune system is incapable of fighting off the virus which can cause the infected person to experience symptoms. Illness and infections become the symptomatic problems that the person must guard against. This syndrome can also be passed down from mother to child. A cure for this disease has not been found. However, there are some treatments that have been successful in the treatment process.

Self-esteem: The regard a person has for themselves on a personal level.

Self-fulfilling prophecy: A prediction or forecast that is spoken and then comes true.

Semantics: The basic meaning of words that relate to the subtleties and relationships found in a language.

Sender: The person that projects a message in order to communicate with another person or group of people.

Shame: The person who has suffered some disgrace or humiliation.

Shock: The body's physical and emotional reaction to extreme emotions.

Social facilitation: Describes how a person responds in a positive way whenever there are others present.

Stage Hogging: Person that speaks out without listening to another person's opinion.

Stress: Feelings associated with the trauma and the event that caused the trauma.

Sublimation: The thought process is refocused to allow the emotions to be redirected in a positive manner.

Suppression: How a person will defer or put off feelings of anxiousness to a time in the future.

Survivor guilt: The feeling that a person has when they feel they could have prevented the death of a loved one in some manner.

Sympathy: Feeling or emotion expressed when you have a compassion for the other person's pain or grief.

Syntax: The way a sentence is assembled in a speech pattern.

Thematic: The first sentence which identifies the main idea of a speech or topic.

Threat: An action to be taken that would cause harm to another person. This usually creates an atmosphere of fear and trepidation.

Tone: The way a voice sounds in terms of inflection. Your tone can be an indicator of the emotions that you are experiencing.

Volume: Soft or loud levels in which a person speaks.

Warmth and Caring: Two qualities noted by Wolfelt which are the ultimate sign of a person that can be both considerate and friendly. These qualities can either be expressed verbally or nonverbally.

Forms of Disposition

Anatomical donation

Anatomical donation has provided much needed educational research to scientists. The deceased person donates his or her body to this research. The medical school or organization that accepts the donation must ensure that the body meets the conditions for this practice. The bodies must be free from emaciation, obesity, extensive burns, mutilation, advanced decomposition, and be free from any history of contagious disease. The decease's age is not a factor. Usually, the body is not used to study the disease that caused the person's death. However, some may request that this be the case. The family must choose either a permanent or temporary donation status. The status of permanent donation gives the organization the right to use the body for an indefinite period of time. The family will not receive the cremains back after it is no longer needed.

If a family chooses, the family can select temporary donation status of the body. Temporary donation status is usually for a period of about 18 months. The cremains are returned to the family after use. This is not the case in a permanent donation. Anatomical donations of organs and tissues are also an option. This option is different from the use of transplants. Anatomical donations do not consider age to be a factor. The person who wishes to make an anatomical donation should make his intentions regarding the donation known to his family members. This prevents any confusion after the person has passed away. The person who makes these arrangements is doing so for the purpose of advancement of education and research. The family members who are cognizant of this desire can best make the decisions regarding their decedent's wishes.

Burial

Burials are performed to dispose the human body in the ground. The form of natural burial is a trend which is growing in popularity. The body is placed in a biodegradable container or shroud. The body is buried in the ground with a tree or shrub planted over the gravesite. This trend differs from the traditional memorial markers made from a granite or marble. Other more traditional forms place the body in a casket which is set into a burial liner or vault. The vault keeps the casket from caving in under the weight of the earth. The vault prevents the flotation of the casket to the top of the water line in case of flood. The vault allows for a smoother ground surface due to the lack of cave-ins around the casket from the earth settlement after a burial.

Cremation

Cremation is an ancient practice for disposal of the body. The body is exposed to extreme heat as high as 1800 degrees in a crematorium. The crematorium may be housed within the funeral home or at another place of business. The law has some specific regulations regarding the cremation of a body. The law states that only one body is allowed to be cremated at any given time. The body is placed in a container consisting of a wood or cardboard material. This container burns with the body. The body is burned in the chamber called a retort. Retorts are fashioned in standardized sizes. This is one reason that a grossly obese person cannot select this option for disposal. The body is burned intact with jewelry, watches, and eyeglasses.

The body is burned intact. However, pacemakers can explode and will have to be removed before the cremation can be performed. An explosion would destroy the cremator. The body is burned for approximately two hours in length. The result of the burn leaves a few bones that are swept into the cremulator. The cremulator grinds up the weakened bones into powder and finer particles. The grinding is accomplished through the use of agitating steel balls. The melted lumps of jewelry, dental fillings, and surgical implants are filtered out at this point. These filtered out particles are buried in a section of the grounds that has been consecrated or set apart from other parts of the cemetery. The remains of the body are referred to by the technical term cremains. However, many people still prefer to use the term ashes.

Duties

Before the funeral

The funeral director should work to build a bond with the family before the funeral. The funeral director should gather the appropriate statistical information used to fill in forms, claims, and in the submission of the funeral's obituary announcement to the officials and to the newspapers. The funeral director must make the arrangements concerning the forwarding and receiving of the deceased for disposition. The funeral director is responsible for explaining the death certificate to the family. The FTC requires that the prices, the price list, the service offerings, and the merchandise are to be explained to the family. The funeral director must also explain and discuss the elements surrounding the disposition options and the requirements of the law regarding the disposition of the body. The funeral director should organize the ceremony and ensure that the participants understand their roles in the funeral service.

The funeral director should organize the transportation for the funeral. This includes providing the proper documentation that is needed for transport. The funeral director is responsible for arranging the clothing of deceased and disposal of the personal items. The funeral director should confer about the cemetery requirements and all the options that are provided. This includes the differences between the funded and the non-funded items. The funeral director is responsible for explaining the revocable and irrevocable funded pre-need arrangements. The funeral director is also responsible for explaining the difference between funded, trust-funded, guaranteed prices, and non-guaranteed prices in pre-need contracts. The funeral director is responsible for organizing the anatomical donations. The body must be released according to the requirements made by the law. The funeral director must also fill out the proper insurance forms for payments to be received for all services and merchandise.

During and after

The funeral director may act as the clergy member during the funeral or explain last minute details. The funeral director must make preparations for the visitation or ceremonial services to be conducted. The funeral director makes decisions regarding the placement of the casket during the services. The director sees to the lightning, floral arrangements, and other personal items that are required. Some personal items may be in accordance to the family's desires, the decedent's life, memorial register, service programs, religious items, and any video or audio equipment. The funeral director should go over any last minute details with the clergyman. The director guides and assists the pall bearers in the procedures. The director arranges the parking for the attendees. The funeral director also oversees the seating of the family and participants during the services

The funeral director oversees the dismissal of the family and the participants after the ceremony. The funeral director is responsible in guiding the cortege to the burial spot. The family must then be returned to designated locations. The funeral director is responsible for overseeing the final disposition of the body. The funeral director must also make sure that the family receives the cremains at the presentation. The director ensures the receipt for the cremains is received from the family. Some directors provide post-funeral counseling as a follow up to the funeral service. This service offers support, education, and resources to the family. This practice allows the coordinator to continue a relationship with the family and ensures further business opportunities when the family is in need of a funeral director. This service can be a marketing tool for the funeral director.

Burial-Transit Permit

The purpose of this document is to provide a legal authorization to those who transport the remains of the decedent. This document is also called the Disposition Permit. Permits can usually be obtained after a death certificate has been presented. The funeral director is responsible to fill out the completed death certificate in full at the local registrar's office. The body can then be transported across the state lines. However, if the body is to be disinterred in another state, the funeral director must obtain a Disinterment Permit and the Burial Transit Permit at the same time. Transportation to another country requires an apostille to be granted by the Secretary of State. All documents may need to be furnished in the language of the country in which the body is to be transported. The translated documents can expedite the process.

Cash advances

The Cash Advance items are paid by the funeral home in the arrangement of a funeral service. The items paid for in advance include flowers, cemetery services, obituary notices, clergy honoraria, and the public transportation. Any applicable service fees also charged by the funeral home must be explained to the consumer before the transactions. In addition, the consumer must be notified if the funeral home receives a discount or a rebate for services purchased. The Federal Trade Commission Funeral Rule holds stipulations that state a consumer has the right to refuse any item that is not desired. The funeral director must provide the consumer with a detailed, itemized listing of all the services and products purchased. Failure to provide this listing is a serious violation of the Funeral Rule. The cost of violations to the Funeral Rule can result in a fine of $10,000.

Medical examiner

The Coroner is the elected officer of a district, region or county who investigates deaths within the community. The Coroner is particularly interested in the investigation of deaths which are unusual or not from natural causes. A Medical Examiner or M.E. is the medical officer, usually appointed, who has received a degree in medicine. The Medical Examiner is a licensed physician with a specialty in pathology or forensic medicine. The advancements in forensic science have caused an expansion in the need for services performed by the Medical Examiner in the community. This position is becoming more prevalent in large cities or more populated regions of the country. In rural areas, the Coroner is still the officer of the local governmental death investigations. The Coroner usually operates as the local funeral director in rural areas.

During the investigation of a death, the Coroner or the Medical Examiner works to determine the time of death, the reason for the death and the mode of death. There are small percentages of deaths that are found to require an autopsy to determine time, cause and manner of death. These facts can usually be determined from observations made at the scene of death and current medical records of the decedent. Neither the Coroner nor the Medical Examiner holds a position as a judicial officer. However, they do have the power of subpoena and to authorize an inquest panel. Each state may have additional functions that are required to be performed. For example, in the state of Georgia, the Coroner is an extension of the sheriff. The Coroner in Georgia can issue warrants, serve process or even act as Sheriff of the county.

Worship types

The Eucharist-Centered Worship is referred to as a Liturgical Worship. This worship has a set structure with defined rituals included. The Blessed Sacrament, Holy Communion, Lord's Supper, and Eucharist are the core element of the worship. Liturgical also means in a more general way the formal ritual of a religious ceremony. This formal ritual is dictated from a religion. One example of this formal ritual is found in the daily Muslim Salats. The Muslim Salats includes five daily ritual prayers. Another formal ritual is found in the Quaker religion as they attend the Quaker Meetings on a regular basis. These are all forms of Liturgical Worship. However, in a structure of worship that is founded upon the basis of Scripture, a Non-Liturgical Worship is the result. The Non-Liturgical Worship is given an order of worship by the individual church or the pastor of that church.

Important terms

Acknowledgement cards: Cards sent out by the family as an expression of gratitude to family and friends that sent flowers, memorials, food, and sympathy to the bereaved members of the family.

Acolyte: Title given to the altar attendant or altar boy. The altar attendant carries the candle or torch that is used during the liturgy. This position receives the highest rating in the minor orders of the ministry, but can be performed by lay members of the congregation.

Aftercare: Follow-up services provided by the funeral director. The coordinator uses this follow up service to keep in touch with the family members. The coordinator may counsel family members during holidays or dates which are associated with the decedent. This coordinator may provide support, education, or additional resources which can assist the family in coping with the loss of their loved one. This is an excellent marketing tool for the funeral service industry as this allows the coordinator to be a part of any future deaths that the family may experience.

Allah: The name of the Muslim God. Translations of this word from the Arabic term to the English word God is somewhat controversial. Some scholars hold fast to the belief that the word "Allah" is an illustration of the uniqueness of the Supreme masculine being. The word, "Allah", is the name given to describe his presence, not his name. The scholars believe that the word "God" does not lend itself to the same meaning as the Arabic word "Allah".

Alternative Container: The receptacle or the box used to place the human remains. This box is made of an unadorned, unlined fiberboard or pressed wood material.

Archbishop: The titled given to show the highest position of a bishop in the Roman Catholic faith. This person works as an administrator over specific territorial regions. The territorial regions are referred to as a diocese or archdiocese. The Greek translation for this word is defined as an overseer or supervisor.

Aron: The name given in Hebrew to refer to a wood container. This box does not have any metal parts.

Artificial Grass: The green mat or carpet covering the earth mound and the grave site area.

Bishop: The administrator placed in charge of a church through an ordination or a Holy Order. This Holy Order implies an authoritative position in the role of administration and in religious matters.

Brethren: Spiritual relationships among a religious congregation.

Brother: A person preparing for ordination in a Roman Catholic Church. The reference can also refer to the pastor or male members of a congregation in a Christian church.

Brotherhood: A social organization of which there are male members.

Canopy/Cemetery Tent: The portable tent which is placed over the grave site. This protective covering protects the funeral service participants from the elements during the committal service.

Cantor: The singer in religious ceremonies who provide assistance to the Clergy, Rabbi, or Priest.

Celebrant: The person who presides over the mass during a Roman Catholic service.

Cemetery: The portion of land that is used for the final resting burial of the deceased.

Chancel: The partitioned off section of the altar used by the clergy and the choir. The partition may be a railing or some type of lattice structure.

Chaplain: The person in a military or other organization who assumes the responsibility for the religious activities that take place. This person can minister to persons of a variety of faiths or denominations. The United States has a House Chaplain and a Senate Chaplain.

Christian Burial Certificate/Permit: The document which provides the certification and authorization in granting permission for a burial in a Roman Catholic Cemetery. This document is also known as Priestly Lines.

Cot: The portable gurney or stretcher that is used for the transportation of those who have died or are in some way incapacitated.

Cross bearer/Crucifer: Person responsible for carrying the crucifix during religious processional ceremonies.

Cross: The Christian symbol or icon used to depict the sacrificial death of Jesus Christ. The empty cross is a symbol of the resurrection of Jesus after his death on the cross.

Crucifix: The Catholic symbol or icon used to depict the image of Christ upon the cross.

Crypt: This is the term used to refer to the compartment within a mausoleum which encases the casket.

Deacon: Elected office in some religious denominations. The elected male or female deacon works as a servant of the religious congregation.

Elder: An older person within the church that is deemed to be wise. The person is usually a non-salaried layman with specific ministerial duties to perform. The terms deacon and elder are terms that are both used to describe this position.

Escort: The leader of a procession or the personnel which accompanies the deceased during transportation.

Eucharist: The consecrated or set apart elements used for the Holy Communion service. This is a service which symbolizes the bread and wine as the body parts of Jesus Christ and in memory of his sacrificial death. This service is also called the Lord's Supper, Divine Liturgy, Mass, or Great Offering.

Final Commendation: The last part of the Catholic ceremony performed in a funeral mass.

Foyer: The entrance hall found within a funeral home or church. This entrance may be called a narthex, a lobby, or a vestibule.

Funeral Liturgy: The mass performed for the funeral of a member of the Roman Catholic Church.

Genuflect: An act that began as the posture of a knight bending on one knee before his king. This gesture has evolved in the Roman Catholic and Anglican religions. The faithful are expected to fall to one knee if they pass before the Blessed Sacrament. The Blessed Sacrament is the wine and bread of the Lord's Supper. The Roman Catholic faith holds to the belief that the Blessed Sacrament has become the body of Christ in its most literal interpretation. In modern times, the Pope has instructed that the faithful should genuflect at the beginning and the end of the ceremony.

Grave Straps: The webbing or ropes used to lower the casket into the grave.

Grave: The hole in which the casket is placed for burial. This is also known in the Hebrew language as the Kever.

Icon: The holy picture made from a mosaic of a painted wood which is found in the Eastern Orthodox religion.

Iconostasis: A screen of separation which acts a divider in the Eastern Orthodox Church.

Imam: Religious leader of a local Islamic congregation.

Islam: The name of the monotheistic religion practiced by those who believe in Allah. This teaching began as teachings of Muhammad in the 7th century AD in Arabia. Muhammad taught from the Qur'an. This religion can be traced back to the Semitic traditions of Abraham.

Memorial Park: The cemetery which has flush to the ground memorial markers for each grave site.

Minister: Authorized or ordained clergyman responsible for the worship services and the care of the congregation. The terms clergy, reverend, or pastor can be used to describe this position.

Muslim: Persons practicing the Islamic faith and who worship Allah.

Nave: The section of the church used for seating the congregation.

Niche: The compartment found inside the columbarium which is used to display the urn.

Prie Dieu: The rail used for by members to kneel upon as they say their prayers. The English translation means prayer rail kneeler.

Qur'an: The writings used by Muhammad in the teachings of the Islamic faith.

Retort: The heating chamber in the crematorium in which the body is heated in the process of cremation.

Rosary Beads: The little beads or jewels on a necklace with a crucifix attached. The beads are used in the recital of the prayers.

Royal Doors: The doors which are found within the middle of the Iconostasis. The doors are used by the ordained clergy to proceed to the altar. The crossing upon the solea in front of the Royal Doors is forbidden.

Sanctuary: The section of church located around the altar. People sit in this location for the worship services.

Scapular: A piece of cloth or medallion worn about the neck of people who practice the Roman Catholic faith.

Sister: Female members of a religious congregation. In the Roman Catholic faith, the nuns are also referred to as sisters. Nuns are the women who take religious vows of dedication for a lifetime of service and sacrifice involving the Lord's work.

Solea: The elevated area of the Eastern Orthodox Church found in front of the Iconostasis or dividing screen.

Tachrichim: The white linen garment used as a shroud for the Jewish decedent.

Tallith: The prayer shawl worn by men of the Hebrew faith. The four corners of the prayer shawl have a symbol called the tzitsit. This symbol represents the 613 commandments given to them by God.

Tomb: The grave or crypt in which the human remains are placed.

Transepts: The wings or small chapels in the main church which are used to perform the wedding or baptismal ceremonies.

Vestments: The garments worn by members of the clergy.

Vigil Lights: The candles or lights placed at the head and the foot of the casket during the Roman Catholic visitation service.

Yarmulke: The Jewish cap worn by men of the Hebrew faith. This is also referred to as a Kippah.

Torts

Torts are civil wrongs which require damages to be recompensed. Torts differ from contracts in that a contract is a promise or agreement made. Penalties can be enforced by the courts when the parties involved in these agreements do not honor their obligations. The courts issue penalties for the breach of contract made. However, torts are generated out of intentional, negligence, and liability. William Prosser deemed that the legality of this term was applicable to a "miscellaneous and more or less unconnected group of civil wrongs." Torts are categorized by the level of intent that takes place. Moral wrongdoing may be corrupt in a societal manner, but may not have regulations which prevent the wrongdoing from occurring. Tort liability is a legal obligation which has been deemed by the court a plausible remedy to the act of wrong doing in civil cases. The damages are required as an answer to the obligation.

Property

Property is a possession in which ownership belongs to an individual or entity. The property can be in the form of a good, product, creative production or resource. Possession of the property assures the owner the privilege to dispense with it as he/she/it sees fit within legal realms. Personal property is often called moveable property and is identified as anything that can be moved. Moveable property can be in the form of money, negotiable, securities, goods, and intangible assets. Real estate property must be transferred by deed to another person or entity. Personal property has no restriction except in the case of vehicles and such. Interest in personal property may be absolute or qualified. The property may be acquired by act of occupancy, by invention, by transfer, by act of law, or by the act of the bequeather.

Business organization types

A **proprietorship** is the most common form of business ownership consists of one owner. The business owner is responsible for all debts and obligations acquired by the business. The income from the business is considered personal income and subject to taxes.

Partnerships are business organizations established between at least two people. In a partnership, general partners have unlimited liability. In a general partnership, all owners may participate in any partnership decisions, creating a decentralized management; limited partnerships may have centralized management, which has proved to be more effective in business operations.

A **corporation** is a business type organization which is considered as a legal person even though it is comprised of numerous persons. There are several types: joint stock companies, for profit, not for profit, and government. The scope of the corporation is determined by the law of the place in which it was formed.

Agency and employment law

An **agency** is an organization with a set of relationships among one or more persons who are authorized to act for the principal of the agency. If the business is a corporation, it is a fictitious person and can only act through agents of the corporation. The principal is liable for any agreements made. The agent makes the agreement based upon instructions given by the principal for negotiations.

Employment law expresses the legal rights of the employees that work for an individual or an entity for monetary gain. Employment law provides some restrictions to these employees as well. Equal opportunity employment is provided. Wages are generally determined by supply and demand. Additionally, other areas of employment are regulated. These areas include: the legal minimum wage; taxes (social security and federal/state income); benefits; disability; and work environment safety (OSHA). Employment laws are provided to protect the employees from unfair labor practices.

Wage and Hour Act

The federal government is responsible for the enforcement of the fair labor laws. One such law is called, "Wage and Hour Act." In 2004 it was reconstructed and renamed. It is now known as the Federal Fair Labor Standards Act. Each state has its own Wage and Hour Act and employment laws. The division responsible for the enforcement of these laws also establishes minimum wage, overtime pay, recordkeeping, and child labor standards. The laws impact the full-time and part-time workers in private sectors, Federal, State, and local governmental agencies. The minimum wage is $7.25 an hour. Overtime pay is required when workers work more than 40 hours in a given week. The rate of overtime is set at a rate not less than one and one-half times their regular rates of pay. Employees who do not receive their wages as stated may contact their state's labor department for assistance.

Commercial paper

Commercial paper is a written agreement. The purpose of the paper is to put into place a written agreement which has a set of provisions and situations under which finances are borrowed by a corporation. This paper acts as a promissory note of repayment of the debt. Commercial paper is issued by large corporations of good credit. These corporations are responsible for borrowing unsecured funds for a short time, usually 90 days, but no more than nine months. Commercial paper is purchased, sold, and traded by individual and corporate investors. The usual purpose is to finance short-term cash flow or purchase inventory. This promise can be in the form of a promissory note, a draft, or a check. The promissory note is simply a promise to pay another party an agreed upon amount as repayment. The promissory note is a negotiable document.

Will, trusts, intestacy, and estate claims

A **will** refers to the legal document which determines how a deceased person's personal property will be divided and dispersed among the beneficiaries and existing creditors. The deceased person must have been over the age of 18 and of sound mind at the time that the will was drafted. A **trust** is a fund which is held by a trustee for specific purposes for a particular person, persons, organization, etc. **Intestacy** is the dispersal of a personal property by the state when a person has died without a will in place. An **estate claim** is one which has been filed against a deceased person's estate to obtain a payment for an outstanding debt or financial obligation.

Important terms

Acceptance: An agreement upon which an offer is established and a signed contract is drawn up.

Accord and Satisfaction: Occurs when a previous contract is executed according to the rights the parties have already negotiated.

Agent: Person who is authorized by the owner or principal to act on behalf of the company or owner when that person is not available.

Alien Corporation: A company incorporated in a foreign country outside the United States.

Answer: Authorized document which outlines the defendant's defense in a legal proceeding.

Antitrust: A law that promotes the competition among companies and corporations.

Appellate Court: The higher court system which is responsible for judicial decisions regarding cases that are appealed.

Arraignment: Court activities involving a person that has been charged with a crime and is given an opportunity to give a plea of guilty or not guilty.

Arrest: The action of police officials when a person is taken into custody.

Assignee: The person to which an assignment or contractual responsibility is given.

Assignment: A contractual agreement where a contract's responsibility or benefit is transferred to another person or entity that was not the original party named in the original contract.

Assignor: The person who initiated the transfer of an assignment.

Authority: Right to act for another person regarding the contractual agreement.

Bailee: Person who receives the personal property without the title to the property in a bailment.

Bailment: Contractual agreement where one individual gives property, but not title, to another person.

Bailor: Individual who gives up the property to another as with the next of kin who delivers the personal effects to the funeral director for the deceased.

Bearer Paper: Instrument or commercial paper that is payable to the person who holds possession of the document.

Bearer: Individual who acquires or gains an instrument of value.

Beneficiary: Person who receives benefit from a bequest of a resource such as life insurance or the property of the decease which has been described in a will.

Bill of Lading: A written agreement between the shipping company and the person who makes the shipment arrangement.

Bill of sale: Authorized written evidence of exchange that documents that a thing of value was sold and verifies the holder's right of possession.

Blackstone's Definition of Law: Quote by Blackstone that states his opinion upon the purposes of the regulations of rules and conduct. These laws guide the right actions as commandments and guide the wrong actions as forbidden or prohibited.

Blank Endorsement: A paper or electronic check which has only the signature of the authorizer with no other descriptive information included.

Board of Directors: Entity of authority elected by the stockholders in order to give the entity the right to make the decisions regarding the management of a company.

Booking: Paperwork portion that documents the arrest made in order to provide the arrested person's identification and to gather facts including fingerprints and photographs of the arrested person.

Bulk Sales Law: State law that requires the notification to all creditors of a property upon the sale of that property as an inventory transference. Not all states require a bulk sales law.

Business Law: Area of law which deals with laws of conducting and operating a business of commerce.

Cashier's Check: A check drawn on the bank's funds which has been signed by the bank officer and is made payable to the bearer of the document.

Certificate of Deposit: Document which the bank issues as certification of receipt of money that also serves as an agreement to pay the funds out in the amount of the sum received.

Certified Check: Authorized check or document which provides the bank as a guarantee on the face amount to be paid to the holder of the document.

Check: A written order to a financial institution to pay upon demand the face amount written upon the order.

Civil Law: Area of law which makes decisions for society through means of provisions regulated by the laws in which people live under.

Close Corporation: Business corporation which is closely held because the corporate stock is held by only a few numbers of people which are usually family members.

Common Law: Area of law which is defined by the courts as binding customs, without the need for written statutes or regulations.

Compensatory Damages: Monetary award given in a loss.

Competency of Parties: Parties involved in forming the contract must have the capacity and reasoning abilities which enable them to understand the terms.

Complaint: Outline of appeal which instigated the suit of legal action.

Consignee: Person who receives goods shipped by a carrier.

Consignor: Person or entity which shipped the goods by carrier.

Contract Assignments: When a contract is transferred to a new owner or the liabilities are transferred to a new responsible party.

Contract: An agreement between two parties to do something or to refrain from doing something. It has three basic components: the offer, the consideration and the acceptance.

Contractual Capability: Portion of the contract which states the needfulness of all parties as being able to meet all obligations of the contract.

Corporation: Legalized entity which operates as a separate and distinct business which provides some protection to the individuals who make up the corporation regarding their intangible responsibility for the business conducted.

Counter Offer: Response to an initial rejection of a contract stipulation by changes in the contract and submitted for the other party's approval/acceptance.

Crime: Deviation from any actions which are not legal.

Criminal Law: Area of law which stipulates and regulates the laws for the legal proceedings in regards to the punishment of wrongdoings committed by persons who have been arrested for a crime.

Defective Agreement: When the contractor or the person who hired the contractor fails to perform or relinquish the agreed upon something of value. This failure causes a Breach of Contract.

Defendant: Person who is accused of wrongdoing by arrest.

Disaffirmance: Decision to refuse or reject a voidable contract.

Discharge: The point in which a contract is terminated because of one of the following reasons: all provisions are fulfilled; agreement; impossibility; acceptance of breach; and operation of law.

Discovery: Gathering and collection of all pertinent information regarding a case before it goes to trial.

Domestic Corporation: Incorporated business which operates within the same state.

Donee Beneficiary: Three party agreement in which party A wants to gift party C with a specific amount. Party A agrees to provide "something" to party B in order to gain payment for party C from Party B. Party C is the Donee beneficiary of this three party agreement.

Draft: Written authorization which documents the order placed by a person or institution to pay a specific sum on a specified date agreed by the authorizing person or company.

Drawee: The financial institution ordered to pay a draft.

Drawer: Person to whom the draft is paid or compensated.

Duress: An action in which force is used as a threat to do harm to a person, family, or belongings.

Employee: Person who works for another in the performance of a specific job for compensation or payment of some kind.

Employer: Person or entity that has hired employees in which they pay for a specific job performance.

Endorsee: Person named on an instrument as the one entitled to receive the endorsement of a negotiable instrument.

Endorsement: Signature on the back of the check or instrument that is cashed or collected upon.

Endorser: Person who signs the instrument indicating reception of funds has been received.

Executed Contracts: Completed contracts once the fulfillment of the stated obligations of a contract have been completed.

Executory Contracts: Uncompleted contracts in which the obligations have not been met.

Existing goods: the term given to the products present at the time of the beginning of the contractual agreement.

Express Authority: Written authority of an agent in a document.

Express Warranty: Verbal or written guarantee of standard or responsibility.

Felony: A crime that is committed which is under the jurisdiction of federal law and constitutes a federal offense.

Fiduciary: The trust or assets between partners in business.

Foreign Corporation: A business which operates in a different state than the one in which it was incorporated.

Formal Contract: The written sealed agreements.

Formalities of a Sale: The requirements that are needed for a contract to be legal.

Fraud: Any illegal action that uses false statements or induces a person to enter contract under false pretenses for a harmful purpose.

Future Goods: Products contracted for in an agreement that will be produced at a future date.

General Agent: Individual who is authorized by a principal to handle all business dealings of a specific kind or at a specific place.

General Partner: Person who is a partner and manages the business either as an individual or a company.

Goods: Moveable products or items that are for sale.

Holder: Individual or entity that possesses or holds a financial instrument.

Identified Goods: Merchandise whereby a negotiated price is determined by the purchaser and the seller.

Illegal Contracts: Any agreement in which a part or the whole does not conform to law violates the law.

Implied Authority: Power of an agent in acting upon the behalf of the principal beyond the written instructions or expressed consent already given.

Implied Contract: Common law created behavior or actions made which suggests the agreement of both parties without the written expression of the agreement.

Implied Warranties: The guarantee which is compelled by law to be honored due to the fact that a thing has been sold.

Independent Contractor: Person or company for work performed at a set fee; the person paid is not a part of the company but works at his own risk.

Injunction: Court order forbidding a particular act.

Intangible Person Property: Ownership of a copyright or stock within a company, having no physical substance.

Judgment: Court decision handed down by a judge in response to litigation.

Judicial System: A network of courts consisting of district, state, and federal jurisdictions which decide if the law has been broken and enforce punishments upon those which have broken the law.

Law: A set of rules which are useful for the control and enforcement of people and organizations within a society.

Liability: The debts and obligations owed by an individual or an entity.

Limited Liability Corporation: Form of business which combines features of a partnership and corporation in order to remove the immensity of the liability from the individual owner. This protects the owner from the loss of all personal property in the event of a law suit.

Limited Partner: Partner who has a liability which is bound by the amount of investment.

Liquidated Damages: Amount of recompense or compensation that can be paid from the assets left in the business that can be sold should a breach of contract be made.

Maker: Individual or entity which executes a promissory note in a contractual agreement.

Malpractice: Professional who commits a breach of contract in his professional work which can either be illegal or cause harm to the person who contracted services.

Merchant: Individual or entity that buys and/or sells goods or products.

Minor: Any individual under legal age or adult consensual age.

Misdemeanor: Any crime punishable by less than one year imprisonment or a by a fine.

Misrepresentation: Act of lying or presenting an illusion that leads people to the wrong conclusion.

Necessaries: The necessities or the things required by humans to live such as food, shelter, and clothing.

Negligence: An individual or an entity which fails to operate in regards to the safety and practically of their clients and customers. Some may deliberately do wrong to others, while some only fail in taking proper precautions to create a safe environment for their customers.

Negotiable Instrument: Written evidence or commercial paper which has a specified amount or value transferable from person to person. Also be used as a credit source.

Negotiation: Actions of deliberation between two individuals, an individual and entity in the transference of ownership regarding a tangible or intangible property.

Nominal Damages: Symbolic gesture of an award by the court with little value, (usually $1.00). This gesture provides the plaintiff with absolution or a release from the obligation.

Novation: Individual under a contract that substitutes another in his place with the agreement of the original contract parties intact.

Offer/acceptance: There must be an offer to consider and an acceptance or approval given before the exchange of something of value in exchange for something of value can take place.

Offer: Act of agreeing to enter into a contract with each other.

Offeree: Person to whom the offer is extended or proffered.

Offeror: Individual who extends or gives the terms of contract.

Order Paper: Document or check that has the words, "payable to the order of", written on it to emphasize the purpose of the financial instrument.

Ordinances: Rules, regulations, and/or laws enacted and enforced by local government.

Parol Evidence Rule: Any evidence which shows that a prior agreement or arrangement made which differs from the written contract is null and void.

Partnership: Two or more persons who enter into a business relationship and accept mutual liability for that business.

Payee: Person or entity to whom any financial instrument is due.

Personal Property: Anything that is not real estate property or real property.

Petition: Complaint or written accusation brought to the court's attention in the case of a wrongdoing resulting in a civil suit.

Plaintiff: Person or entity that is accusing another in a civil law suit.

Price: the term given to describe the value on goods, personal property, real property, etc. as described in the contract.

Principal: Responsible party in a business who hires another to negotiate the business transactions.

Private Corporation: Non-government business operation owned by several individuals.

Process: The summons or paper which gives notification to a defendant in regards to the impending litigation which requires a formal response such as appearance in court

Promissory Estoppel: Legal prevention of the promisor from withdrawing his promise after the promisee comes to harm after acting upon the promise made by the promisor.

Promissory note: Financial instrument which has a stated obligation of a promise to pay.

Public Corporation: Company that conducts governmental functions within a community.

Punitive Damages: Court awards which are given as chastisement to the defendant.

Qualified Endorsement: Endorser who has accepted limited liability.

Ratification: Process of making something valid after it has already occurred as in the case of a confirmation or a previously unauthorized adoption.

Real Property: Land or buildings and structures upon that land.

Reciprocity: The mode of exchange in which transactions take place between individuals as equals. This also refers to the state's ability to extend the same privileges to a license holder in another state as to the license holder in its own domain or region.

Rejection: Refusal to agree or accept a contract's terms.

Remedies for Breach of Contract: The judicial system controls and makes judgments regarding any violations of contracts. Insignificant problems may be resolved without involvement from the courts.

Replevin: this refers to the recovering of possessions or property that has been lost.

Rescission: Voiding or cancellation of an agreement.

Restrictive Covenant: Deed limits for the use of property or the prohibiting of certain activities of use of property.

Restrictive Endorsement: Stated use which has been written removing all chances for the possibility of using the endorsement for any other purpose than what is stated.

Revocation: Removal or cancellation of authority of one making a promise in regards to a financial instrument.

Rules and Regulations: Laws and enforcement of those laws by a governing agency.

Sale: Exchange of value of a good or service for monetary gain or some other benefit.

Secured Claim: The pledging of property for the settlement of a debt.

Service Contracts: Agreement involving services rather than goods.

Shareholders: this title refers to the stockholders or persons who represent the owners of a corporation who own all the stock of the corporation.

Sherman Antitrust Act: Legislation preventing one corporation from restraining trade of another corporation in an effort to promote healthy competition.

Silent Partner: Individual who only provides capital for investment purposes and takes no active part in running the business.

Simple Contract: Straight written, oral, or implied upon agreement between two parties.

Sole Proprietorship: Business which is owned by an individual.

Special Agent: Authorized person or company to perform business acts for a principal.

Special Endorsement: Person in whom payment is made.

Special Performance: Court order decision involving the party who breached a contract to fulfill the contract.

Stare Decisis: A precedent of previous court decisions which is used as a guide for later decisions by another court.

Statues: Acts of legislature which are known as laws.

Statute of Fraud: Certain kinds of contracts are to be in a written format.

Statute of Frauds: Law that states enforcing a contract can only happen with the contract or agreement which has been written.

Statute Of Limitations: Law that sets a time limit on when a criminal action can be brought to court legally.

Subchapter S Corporation: Tax law that allows shareholders to be taxed as a partnership rather than as a corporation with the added benefit of not losing their corporate standing.

Termination: The end of the contract.

Transfer of Risk: Risk management technique that reassigns the financial risk from one party to another party. One example is when insurance is purchased. The financial loss risk from the insured goes to the insurer in the transfer.

Transfer of Title: The signed document registered to one person showing ownership is reassigned to another person for ownership purposes.

Undue Influence: Action of a person in using overt pressure upon another without threat of harm.

Unenforceable Contract: Improper legal form of an agreement that the courts cannot require to be fulfilled due to its form.

Uniform Commercial Code: Regulation which provides a consistent and uniform regulation of state laws across the country as they apply to commerce.

Unilateral Contract: Agreement for exchange of payment for service only when the service has been done or completed.

Usurious: this refers to the charging of an exorbitant rate of interest which goes above a fair rate.

Valid Contract: Documents which are described as legally enforceable agreements.

Void Contract: Agreement that is annulled with no legal recourse.

Voidable Contract: Enforceable agreement with the provision of circumstances which can cause one or the other party to set the contract aside.

Warranties: A written or implied statement that states that a provision in a contract is true. Usually this promise is made by a manufacturer or a seller to indicate responsibility for any losses the consumer may incur due to product defects of goods sold.

Guaranteed contract

The guaranteed contract provides a binding agreement for pre-paid funeral services. The funeral merchandise and services are pledged ahead of time. Then, upon the time of need the funeral offers these services and merchandise as agreed upon. The amount of the actual funeral service cannot go over the agreement price regardless of any inflation from the date of contract to date of need. State laws regulate the negotiations of these contracts. These arrangements do not necessarily have to be paid for at the time of the pre-planning arrangement. However, some funeral homes use the money to purchase insurance policies. This purchase makes it easier for the consumer to make monthly payments until the policy is paid in full. This arrangement provides the consumers a cost savings because the services and products are less expensive at the time of purchase than in latter years.

Forwarding the remains

Forwarding the Remains is a process in which one funeral home collects the decedent and transports the decedent to another funeral home in another city or state. The fees for this service must be a part of the General Price List when the service is offered. The omission of this fee on the General Price List could result in a violation of the Funeral Law. The practice of embalming the body may or may not be necessary. The General Price List (GPL) must reflect the inclusion of embalming with the words "if relevant" or "if necessary" included next to the word embalming. Families may opt to call a body shipping service or may call the receiving funeral home to retrieve the body. This allows the family to save the cost of having two funeral homes involved. These options can be a significant cost savings for the family.

Truth in Lending Law

The Federal Truth in Lending Law is an act that involves the legal responsibility of those who extend credit and charge finance fees. Any funeral home which extends credit must comply with this law. This means that the funeral director must discuss the sales contract with the consumer. The discussion includes: cash price of the service/merchandise; down payment amount; difference between down payment and cash price; any other charges of things included in financed amount; charges not part of the finance charge; balance; amount of deductible; unpaid balance and deductible difference; finance charge total; deferred payment price including the total of the cash price plus advances or finance charges; annual percentage rate; number of payments, rate of payments; dates of payments; penalty charged for late payment; security and descriptions; and computation methods on unearned portions of finance charge in event of prepayments.

Government death benefits

There are a number of death benefits provided by the government. Social Security provides a lump sum benefit. This sum equals $255. This amount is paid upon the death of an insured worker. This amount goes to an eligible widow or widower or child of the deceased. The application for this benefit must be made within two years of date of death. In addition, the Social Security Administration will assist the families left behind. The assistance may take the form of monthly payments paid to dependents of the deceased. However, the checks that are received directed to the decedent for the month that the person dies should not be cashed. These monies should be returned to the Social Security Administration. A phone call to this agency should be made to clarify the actions that the bereaved family should take at the time of their loved one's death.

VA death benefits

The Veteran's Death Benefit provides burial arrangements for eligible veterans and also to an eligible veteran's wife, husband, widow, widower, minor children and disabled unmarried adult children. Veterans must be a veteran of any war or retired or discharged from service due to a disability received in line of duty to qualify for this benefit. The benefit must be filed within two years of interment of the deceased. The Veteran's Administration will supply flags to drape the casket for veterans who were retired or discharged under conditions that were not dishonorable from armed forces. The VA will also supply headstones or markers for any honorably discharged veteran. The National Cemetery burial is reserved for active duty and honorable discharged veterans who were awarded decorations such as the medal of honor, Distinguished Service Cross, Distinguished Service Medal, Silver Star, Purple Heart or who was an elected government official, a Chief Justice, a Class 1 Chief, a 5USC 5312 or a 5 USC 5313 officer.

Meeting terms of contract

The funeral director should refer all questions of a legal nature to the client's attorney or a legal professional. The funeral director should obtain and keep on file signatures and credit agreements. All parties involved in any agreement or contract should keep copies of the arrangements. Oral understandings should be written down and signed. All the parties involved should have access to a document which clearly states the responsibilities and financial obligations arranged within the agreements and contracts whether oral or written. A system should be in place which allows legal documents to be stored and retrieved easily. The director should be able to explain estate claims; final disposition of express contracts; implied contracts and quasi-contracts, applicable disclosures and requirements of warranties; embalming, cemetery, crematory and funeral home payment policy; and funeral contracts. The funeral home director should remain in compliance with all federal, state and local laws.

Types of contracts include:
- Irrevocable Contracts: Pre-need contract or agreement which cannot be cancelled or retracted.
- Non-guaranteed: Pre-need contract or agreement which furnishes the funeral home and the consumer with an agreed upon amount that is pre-paid for the funeral service. This pre-payment goes toward the purchase of services and products. However, this arrangement does not set the costs of the services and products at the time of death. Family members will need to pay those extra costs at that time.
- Revocable Contracts: Pre-need contract can be cancelled at any time prior to death. A full reimbursement of monies will be refunded in accordance with state law.

Important terms

Abatement: Reduction of an inheritance when the actual assets do not cover the full bequest.

Actual Custody of the Body: Physical possession of the dead body.

Ademption: An act similar to that of a revocation of a will allowing for the exception that at the time of execution of the will, the property is no longer owned by the testator.

Administrative Agency: The appointed group operating within the government to organize and put into operation particular legislation.

Administrative Law: this is the term used for the rules and regulations of each governmental agency responsible for the legislation, orders and decisions of said agency and the enforcement of those laws.

Administrator: this is the term used for the person in charge of an estate placed in that position by the court.

Administratrix: this term refers to the title given to a female person placed in charge of an estate by the court.

Agent Driver: this is the title given to the person who is supervised by the funeral director. The driver's actions come under the responsibility of the funeral director in this case.

Apprentice: this is the intern, resident or trainee who is in the process of learning to become a funeral director; an embalmer. The licensed funeral director or embalmer is held liable and accountable for the actions of the trainee.

Bequest: this term is given to a gift of personal property by the statement of a will.

Body Parts: this term refers to the organs, tissues, eyes, bones, arteries, blood, bodily fluids, and other portions of a human body used for transplantation and donated under the Uniform Anatomical Gift Act. A donation not revoked by the donor, becomes irrevocable and does not require the consent of others upon the death of the donor.

Brain Death: this is the term given to describe the point at which there is no activity in the brain as indicated by a flat line on the EEG monitoring screen.

Building Code: this refers to the regulations which restrict the construction, the maintenance, and/or the appearance of a building.

Cadaver: this refers to the dead human body which is used for scientific study and research labs.

Case Law: this refers to the decisions of the court which have set precedence and principles regarding previous cases that apply to the current case.

Clinical Death: this refers to the legal death marked by no vital signs and recorded by a doctor.

Codicil: this refers to an alteration or an adding to a will which is executed or carried out with as formal terms as the will itself.

Common Carrier: this refers to an airplane, train, taxi or other vehicle which is used for the transport of persons or freight when the passage for that transportation has been paid.

Common Law: this is the term given to an unwritten system of law which is based on judicial precedents or customs and not on current legislation.

Constructive Custody: this is the term that refers to the controlling disposition of property despite the physical possession of someone else. For example, the funeral director has constructive custody of the deceased because he/she controls the final disposition of the body.

Corpse: this refers to a dead human body that has not completely decomposed.

Crime: this term refers to an act that is legally wrong and violates a law such as treason. The charges resulting may be tried as a felony or misdemeanor as deemed appropriate by law enforcement.

Creditor's Claim: this term refers to the process of collecting upon a debt from the person's estate after the person has died.

Custodian: this is the title given to the person in charge who has a duty to perform a legal protective role over a possession. For example, the funeral director is the custodian of the dead human body when it is removed until final disposition.

Death: this refers to all absence of life, vital signs and/or brain activity within a person.

Degree of Kindred: this refers to level of kinship or relationship as in each generation is considered one degree removed from the decedent.

Devise: this refers to the gift of real estate as stated in a will.

Devisee: this refers to the person that is the inheritor of real estate left in the will.

Disinterment/Exhumation: this refers to the act of removing a body from its burial or resting place.

Doctrine of Stare Decisis: this refers to the policy and actions taken by courts in following rulings based on previous rulings or precedents already set.

Embalmer: this is the title given to the licensed professional who removes blood from the body and replaces it with preservative fluid, disinfects the body, and prepares the body for burial.

Eminent Domain: this is the term given to reservation of power held by the government in acting upon the taking of private real property for public usage after a reasonable compensation has been paid for the property.

Escheat: this is the term given when the decedent has no heirs and the legacy reverts to the state as unclaimed.

Estate: this is the term given to the decedent's property at the time of death.

Ethics: this is the term used to refer to a system of standards based on moral principles which are traditionally adhered to by a specific group.

Executor: this is the title of the person appointed by the deceased within the confines of the will and who is placed in charge of distributing the deceased's estate according to the will.

Executrix: this is the title of the female person appointed by the deceased within the confines of the will and who is placed in charge of distributing the deceased's estate according to the will.

Federal Trade Commission: this is the title given to the governmental agency known as the FTC which supervises the fair competition and ethical practices of industries within the U.S. Some of the unethical practices can be in the form of false advertising, trade restraints, or other unfair practices that gives the companies unfair advantages.

Fetal Death: this term refers to the death of a fetus before it is born into the world.

Funeral Director: this is the title given to the licensed individual who embalms dead human bodies and/or who operates a business for the purpose of disposition of dead human bodies in the funeral industry.

Funeral Establishment: this is the title given to the place where dead human bodies are prepared for the custom rites and for final disposition or burial.

Guardian: this term refers to the person appointed by the judicial system as one who acts as a custodian over a person who does not have legal capacity to take care of himself such as a mentally disabled person or a child.

Heir: this is the title given to the person(s) who receives a bequest or who is entitled to the bequest by law regarding the deceased's estate.

Householder: this is the title given to the individual who owns or controls the house where a death happened.

Inheritance: this refers to the estate which is bequeathed to heirs after the reading of a will.

Insolvent Estate: this refers to a debt encumbered estate where the value does not exceed the debt that was left owing by the deceased.

Intestate: this refers to the person that dies without a will in place.

Intestate Succession: this refers to the person that inherits personal or real property because a will was not written.

Interstate: this refers to the condition of being between states or among states.

Intrastate: this refers to the condition of being within a single state.

Inventory (in Probate): this refers to the itemization and valuation of the estate by an agent of the estate for an appraisal of worth.

Justice of Peace: this refers to the title given to a magistrate or a civil appointed government official who performs the duties required of him or her.

Kin: this refers to the people in which you have blood relation.

Law: this refers to the rule or ordinance which can be enforced by an authoritative body or governmental agency.

Legacy: this term refers to the estate left by a decedent.

Legatee: this refers to the person who receives a bequest or inheritance under the stipulations of a will.

Liability: this refers to a legal responsibility regarding the circumstances surrounding a wrongful or accidental act caused by negligence.

Lien: this refers to the legal claim a person or organization has upon personal or real property due to debts that are owed to them.

Live Birth: this refers to the delivery of a living breathing baby at the end of a pregnancy.

Livery: this refers to a uniform worn by a driver in hired out automobiles such as limousines.

Malpractice: this term refers to a professional who commits an act of negligence either willfully or ignorantly that causes injury to someone under their care.

Medical Examiner/Coroner: this refers to the person who investigates the cause of death of a person to determine whether it is by accident, suicide or homicide. This professional can pronounce the death and issue a death certificate when there is no medical doctor present at the time of death.

Mental Anguish: this term is given to suffering resulting from sustained, painful emotion caused by distress, intense grief, or severe anxiety.

Morgue: this is the term used to refer to a holding place for dead, unidentified human bodies until identified or until the final disposition is arranged.

Moral Turpitude: this refers to a felonious type of crime which is willful and purposeful in nature.

Mortuary Law: this refers to the system of laws which deals with the organizations that perform final dispositions and their operation in the disposal of the dead. Mortuary jurisprudence or the Funeral service law is also a way to refer to this law.

Mutilation: this refers to the defacing of an object or the disfigurement of a corpse. Embalming without permission is considered mutilation because it alters the body from the original condition which is expected.

Negligence: this refers to the professional who does not perform up to the standard expected and results in harm. This act can also be an omission of an action that a reasonable person would do to safeguard customers or property from harm.

Nuisance: this term refers to when the owner of a property uses that property in a way that gets in the way of or interferes with another property owner.

Nuisance in Fact: this term refers to the actions which has the potential to become a nuisance.

Nuisance Per Se: this is the term given when an action or thing is a nuisance all the time, or impinges on the civil rights or societal morals of a person and/or can be harmful to persons or property.

Nuncupative: this is the term given to the spoken wishes of a dying person in front of witnesses which imparts the person's will and is later written down.

Ordinance: this is the term given to the legislation of a city or public township which is not covered by federal or state laws and is enforceable by the local laws.

Outrageous Act: this is the term that is committed without any discretion of proper behavior or thought.

Per Capita: this term refers to the inheritances and the estate divisions where all equal degree parties receive equal parts of the inheritance.

Personal Service Contract: this term refers to the agreement between persons for assistance that requires a private knowledge, special skills and the assurance of privacy.

Per Stirpes: this term refers to the degree of kinship which is used when an inheritance is divided among the beneficiaries of a deceased beneficiary.

Personal Representative: this refers to the title given of an executor or administrator of an estate.

Police Power: this refers to the authority of a civil, state, or federal governmental power in making and enforcing the laws for the benefit of its citizens.

Precedent: this refers to the previous judicial ruling of similar cases decided on in a court of law.

Pre-funded Arrangements: Arrangements which include the services previously agreed upon and previously paid.

Preparation Room: this refers to the place in which the embalming and disinfecting of the deceased takes place.

Pre-Planned Arrangements: Arrangements and products are previously selected without the pre-purchase of the services and merchandise.

Private Carriers: this is the term given to refer to the transporters that are contracted for specific transportation.

Probate: this refers to the action taken in the verification of a will.

Probate Court: this refers to the type of court which handles estate matters regarding the will.

Quasi Contract: this refers to a court applied fictitious contract for a mentally disabled person or a decedent where there is no agreement between persons set. This usually takes place after undue enrichment has occurred.

Quasi-Property Theory: this refers to the accepted legal status of a corpse and the final disposition rights that pertain to this status.

Soldiers and Sailors Will: Disposition of personal property of a soldier or sailor in a verbalized statement or nuncupative will.

Solvent Estate: Assets of an estate exceed the debts left owed by the deceased.

Statute: A law or ordinance set by a legislative body.

Statutory Law: Law created by legislature that is written out, unlike the common law or case law which is implied.

Testate: State or condition of having a will.

Testator: Title of the person who has a will.

Testatrix: Female person who has a will in place.

Tort: Civil wrong done to another as in the case of a breach of contract.

Trust Account: An account for the purpose of financially providing the survivors a way of paying for the funeral expenses. This money is usually placed in an account with a funeral home.

Transfer Remains: The first time a body is moved from the location of death to the funeral home or other designated location. This is also referred to as a First Call or a Removal.

Transfer Vehicle: Automobile used for transportation of the body to the funeral home or designated location. Law enforcement usually has the jurisdiction over the scene of death. However, in usual circumstances, it is the Coroner who has jurisdiction over the dead body. Vehicles that have a dead body inside are usually moved out of the public view for dignity's sake. This is usually a joint decision made by law enforcement and the Coroner.

Trustee: Person committed to handling the funeral arrangements on behalf of the family and the person who has the legal right to property in trust for another's benefit.

Uniform Anatomical Gift Act: The UAGA or the legislation which covers the donation of bodies and body parts to scientific research and study purposes.

Uniform Probate Code: Model by which all states achieve homogeny in probate proceedings.

Unsecured Claim: Assertion or claim which is not accompanied by the pledge of property for debt.

Vital Statistics: Data that is gathered and recorded concerning marriages, deaths, births, adoptions, and stillbirths.

Volunteer Driver: Person not under direct supervision of the funeral director during a funeral service.

Will: Written statement or legal document of a person dispersing all personal wealth to beneficiaries which is effective upon the death of the person.

Whole Life Insurance: Coverage for a death loss which lasts the lifetime of the person insured.

Working Capital: Actual cash flow that can be derived when you subtract the value of current assets from current liabilities.

Zoning Ordinance: Law within a municipality which permits and restricts commerce to particular regions of the municipality or city.

Funeral Service Merchandising

Casket construction

A casket is a box or container which is designed to hold a dead human body for purpose of a burial or entombment. The casket provides a protective element regarding the burial or entombment of the body. Likewise, a casket can be used in the cremation process. The casket is usually made of metal, wood, fiberglass, plastics or a combination of the above materials. The parts of the casket include: the eye, rim flange, roll (cove, puffing), cap bracket & cover, header, header flange, crown, pie, rim/ogee, top body molding, corner hardware, arm (lug, ear), base molding, bar, head panel, pillow, hinge skirt, extendover, and an overlay/overthrow. There are a variety of styles of caskets that may be purchased. The caskets that are available can be intricately detailed or of relative simplistic structure.

Opening styles

The opening styles of caskets include: lift panels, hinged panels, full hinge panels, diagonal couch, half couch, three-quarter couch, full couch, half couch perfection, full couch perfection, eternity bed, priest casket, and reverse hinge. The lift panel style is panels that are not hinged to the ogee. However, the panel does rests on the ogee. Hinged panels are head and foot panels which are hinged to the ogee. Full hinged panels are like the hinged panel in structure; however, the head and foot panels are raised to view the body. The diagonal couch is a panel that is cut. This cut provides a division of the head panel and foot panel at a 45 degree angle instead of the usual 90 degree angle. This position allows about ¾ of the right side and ½ of the left side of the body to be viewed at one time.

The half couch allows the upper half of the decedent to be viewed. The three-quarter couch allows ¾ of the upper portion of the body to be viewed. The full couch allows the whole lid to be raised and the ogee is hinged so that the interior can be displayed. The half couch perfection allows the ogee and head panel to be styled as one piece and the upper half of the body is viewed. The full couch perfection allows the entire lid to be raised and has a foot panel to cover the lower half of the decedent. The eternity bed has no inner foot panel but a blanket is used to cover the lower half of the decedent. The priest casket's whole lid may be removed so the full body can be viewed. The reverse hinge is made so the left side of the body is viewed.

Outer burial containers

The outer burial containers hold the casket and are known generally as vaults or grave liners. These containers support the earth load and are made of wood, concrete, metal, polymer and fiberglass. The support of the earth load is necessary so that any heavy equipment used to maintain the grave or to dig graves nearby do not crush the casket. Vaults have a sealant quality and therefore limit the deteriorating effects of other elements. Air seal, aka Bell Dome Seal, creates an air pressure which keeps water from rising to the casketed remains. Top seal uses tongue-in-groove along with an epoxy to maintain the integrity of the casket. A double seal is used with an epoxy along with the air pressure method to keep the casket fastened. Gasket seal or end seal is an old fashioned method which uses a rubber gasket as the closing sealant.

Fundamental merchandising

Merchandising is the business of buying and selling some commodity for a profit. Sales are carefully monitored to ensure that a balance is maintained regarding overhead, cost of product, practices that produce the desired profit based on human needs and the market, competition, regional pricing and business ethics. A sound plan regarding the probable income and expenses for the coming year should be addressed. The funeral director needs to have at least a basic rudimentary knowledge of selling merchandise in order to succeed. However, some directors choose to employ effective sales people to perform this task for them. Merchandising can include an effective website that brings the funeral home closer to its public and has the advantage of providing an interactive section available for the consumer. This section can include prayer cards, pre-need forms, obituaries, or other tools for the consumer's use.

Important terms

Air Tray: A wooden plate with a cardboard covering that can be used as a casket for transportation of the deceased.

Alternative Container: A receptacle which is non-metal and composed of cardboard, compressed wood or canvas or other material, with no ornamentation or fixed interior lining. The container serves the purpose of holding human remains according to the FTC.

Apron: The lining attached to the foot panel and the overlay of the casket.

Arm: The piece of the handle which attaches to the bar of the casket.

Average: The mathematical equation achieved by adding a group of numbers and dividing the total of that sum by the number of units or mean.

Bail Handle: Single unit handle where the bar, arm and lug are one solid structure.

Bar: Part of the handle which is used to carry the casket by the pallbearers in a funeral service.

Base Molding: The ornamentation which is on the lowest edge of the body panels of a casket.

Bed: The inside part of the casket where the deceased rests or is laid.

Bi-Unit Pricing: A mode of pricing which separates services from casket prices in the costs for a funeral.

Body: Part of the casket which is comprised of the top body molding, body panel, base molding and the bottom of the structure.

Body Lining: The material which drapes or hangs over the interior of the casket.

Body Panels: The shell or the sides and the ends of the casket.

Broadcloth: A type of material which has a smooth lustrous appearance and has a dense thread count made of cotton, silk, rayon, woolen or worsted fabric.

Bronze: A type of metal which is comprised of 90% copper and 10% tin or zinc and is used in the making of the casket.

Brushed Finish: The metal surface purposely scratched and then finished off with a high gloss coat to create this appearance.

Cap: The upper most portion of the casket including the ogee, crown, pie and header.

Cap Panel: The focal point of the interior referred to as the panel which fills the crown of the casket.

Cash Advances: Those items which are paid in advance by the funeral home on behalf of the client. These items can include: accommodations, cash disbursements, and cash advances for a service or merchandise.

Cash Discount: A reduction of cost due to prompt payment within contract guidelines.

Casket Rack: A display of two or three caskets one upon the other used for the viewing of different styles of caskets.

Casket Stand: A support used for displaying a casket in the display room.

Cast Bronze: The melted bronze poured into a mold and allowed to cool which is used to make parts for the casket.

Cast Hardware: The fixtures of a casket made in one piece by pouring molten metal in a mold and then cooled to fashion into the correct shape.

Church Truck: A holder with wheels for the casket used for moving the casket with relative ease.

Combination Case: A transfer particleboard box with a cardboard tray used to satisfy air shipping regulations for transportation of the body.

Combination Unit: Two or more items that are intended to be used as one casket and burial receptacle for a single decedent.

Consecutive Method: A merchandising method of displaying items in increasing or decreasing values for the purpose of sales.

Consignment: A sale in which the owner of an item gives it to another for custody or to sell the item.

Consumer Value Index: The wholesale cost of an item that has been divided by its retail price.

Copper: A metal which has the ability to turn green in color through oxidization; before that it is a reddish-brownish-gold color.

Copper Deposit: The copper ions that have been joined by electrolytic processes in the making of the copper core casket.

Corner: Optional casket hardware attached to each corner of the casket.

Crepe: A type of thin, crinkled fabric which can be from silk, cotton, rayon, or wool material.

Crinkled Finish: An exterior finish treatment that is applied to a less expensive casket where a metal is covered with a material that has a wrinkled effect.

Crown: The portion of the casket which extends from rim to rim on the upper most part of the cap.

Crushed Interior: The lining material placed on a metal form with weights added. Then the material is steamed and attached to a suitable upholstery backing material to form the interior of the casket.

Demonstration Group: The marketing design where three or four caskets are arranged for the purpose of educating the persons choosing a casket about casket construction.

Direct Lighting: The arrangement of lights that highlights a group or an object with a direct beam of light.

Direct Selection Room Procedure: The way that a funeral director stays with the persons choosing a casket all the way through the selection process.

Doeskin: A type of fabric which is durable with suede like nap on one side that is used as a material for the casket.

Dome: A type of vault which can support the weight of heavy equipment or earth and has the unique design of being able to trap air in the upper portion when it is placed in position.

Elliptic: A shape of the ends of the casket which are half-circles instead of squared shapes.

Embossed: The imprinted designs in the casket that can either be pressed into the metal, or raised designs within the metal.

Extendover: The part of the interior used for the visual effect that reaches over the top body molding of the casket.

Ferrous Metal: A type of metal that has iron content.

Fiberglass: A type of construction material made of glass filaments in resins that is a versatile material.

Fixed Multiple: A straight line equation in which the cost is multiplied by a constant factor.

Flaring Square: The design style of a casket which has a smaller bottom than the top and the sides and ends swoop out forming the top.

Flat Finish: The matte or dull finished surface.

Fluorescent Lighting: A type of lighting using fluorescent bulbs which can be a less expensive lighting option that is harsh on the eyes.

Foot-candle: The amount of energy used by one candle lighting a one foot distance space in an area.

Foot Panel: The inside part of a casket located at the footer section of the cap above where the feet of the decedent rest inside.

Functional Pricing: A pricing design where the list is determined by the purpose of the item in use as a utility or service, rather than the design of an itemized listing.

Galvanized: A rust-resistant coating of zinc applied to steel.

Gasket Channel: The place on the cut top of a gasket casket that holds the gasket and seals the space between the foot and head caps of the casket.

Gauge: A measure of steel thickness which is the number of sheets it would take to make a one inch thickness.

Gimp: The fold of a piece of material such as metal, cloth, or plastic which covers the area where the roll is attached inside the panel within the casket.

Graduated Recovery: The occurrence in which the return on an investment is realized by a sliding scale profit of each item of merchandise.

Grave Box: The outer receptacle with a one or two piece lid which contains the body of the deceased.

Hammertone: A type of paint that makes the metal appear as if it has been struck by a hammer to form an indentation.

Hardware: The items attached to the outside of the casket such as handles, bars, settings, and other ornamental pieces.

Head Panel: The part of the casket interior that is situated inside the head cap of the container.

Hermetically Sealed: The type of lock that shuts out air, water, and any other environmental influence.

Hinge Cover: The skirt that hides from view the hinges and normally extends into the roll as part of the lining of the casket.

Incandescent Lighting: Type of light that uses a heated filament for a light source.

Indirect Lighting: A reflected light that is not intrusive.

Indirect Selection Room Procedure: The process of allowing persons choosing a casket to roam about without the presence or guidance of the funeral director.

Inner Panels: The functional or ornamental panel covering the foot and possibly the head of the full couch casket's interior.

Itemization: The pricing design where everything is listed separately on the bill.

Laminates: The materials which are typically made from wood and are layered forming a whole panel.

Linen: A type of fabric made from flax which has a sheen and is cool to wear in warm weather.

Linen Weave: A certain look to a fabric or paper made to look like linen.

Lug: Part of the handle that attaches to the casket.

Masselin: Paper upholstery used as backing in a casket.

Median: The middle number in a list where there are as many numbers above as below.

Merchandise Value Ratio: The comparison of the relationship between the wholesale cost of an item or service and the total cost of that item or service.

Mode: The number which reoccurs most often within a list of numbers.

Non-ferrous Metal: Metal which does not contain iron.

Octagon: The shape of an eight-sided casket body panel.

Ogee: The rim or the S-shaped molding on the casket cap.

Ogee Flange: The rim flange or the part of the rim that comes into contact with the casket body.

Pie: The fishtail or the downward slope like a piece of pie and is found at each end of the crown on the top of the casket.

Plastic: The synthetic or organic materials used to make a multitude of products.

Plastic Extrusion Molding: The way plastic is shaped through a process where the material is injected into a mold.

Plated: The electrolytic process of depositing ions of one type of metal on to another type of metal causing the electrons to be shared.

Plush: A type of thick fabric with a nap larger than 1/8th inch which is described as luxurious.

Plywood: The sheets of wood attached to each other with their grains perpendicular with an odd number of sheets used so the grains of the front and back are aligned with each other.

Polished: A high gloss finish that has a shiny or burnished appearance.

Polymer: A durable compound with heavy molecular structure.

Pressed Board: A particle board made from pieces of wood glued together to make sheets.

Quantity Discount: The occurrence where only a certain amount of an item is ordered at one time.

Quartile: The division of a total whereby each equal part is ¼ of the entire whole.

Range: The upper and lower limits of a sequence of figures or numbers.

Rebate: Monetary return of payment already made.

Roll: The cove, the puffing, or the portion of the lining which runs around the inside rim and around the cap panel of the casket.

Satin: A shiny fabric that is smooth to touch and has a dull finish on the backside of the fabric.

Sales Frequency: A set time frame in which the number of times a sale in a set price range occurs.

Sectional: Six to eight concrete slabs which are used for the lining of the grave.

Selected Hardwood: The Salix or the several different types of wood making up the different parts of the casket.

Semi-Gloss: The slightly shiny finish of a surface.

Semi-Tailored: A visual effect found in a combination of styles of casket interior.

Shell: The body of the casket and the lid or the cap of the casket.

Shirred Interior: Fabric used within the casket that has gone through a sewing process which makes the fabric to appear as if it had parallel lines.

Stainless Steel: Metal alloy designed to resist rust used in the making of a casket.

Stamped Hardware: Casket fixtures that are pressed out by hydraulic process rather than molded process.

Stationary Bar: Type of handle that remains in the same place without moving.

Steel: Metal alloy of iron and carbon used in the making of a casket.

Sundry Items: Assorted merchandise that complements the funeral home's services.

Swing Bar: The type of handle on a casket that moves.

Tailored Interior: The fabric of the interior that is tightly drawn over the surfaces.

Threaded Fastener: A screw-type used in the making of the casket.

Throw: The visual effect consisting of an overlay that covers the foot panel of the casket.

Tip: The ornamental part of the handle that covers the open ends of the casket.

Top Body Molding: The body ledge or the molding at the upper edge of the body panels of the casket.

Top Body Molding Flange: The body ledge flange or the part on the horizontal edge of the body ledge that holds the gasket for sealing.

Transfer Container: The box that encases the casketed remains as protection during transport of the body.

Tufted Interior: An interior style that has padding between the inner lining and the outer lining with stitching that makes either a carriage tufting or a biscuit tufting.

Twill Weave: A textile weaver's work in crossing threads over one another to create a look of diagonal lines.

Unfinished Box: A casket that has no ornamentation and no fixed lining, but a plain appearance.

Unit Pricing: Pricing design which gives one price as a package deal for service and merchandise sold.

Urn: Container used to hold cremated remains to be given to the family.

Urnside: Design of a body panel on a casket that has the shape of a vase with a pedestal.

Vault: Sealable grave liner used for disinterment.

Velvet: Smooth, shiny fabric that has a nap on one side.

Vertical Side Square: The body style of a casket that has sides and bottom at 90 degree angles.

Wood Veneer: A thin sheet of superior wood glued to inferior wood to give the appearance of a finer piece of wood.

Wood Wool: Shavings or clippings from wood.

Wrought Bronze: Rolled up sheets of bronze metal.

Wrought Copper: Rolled up sheets of copper metal.

Ziegler Case: The sealed case that can be used as a shipping container or as an insert into a casket.

Accounting principles

Accounting is a methodology of finances where financial information is used to keep systematic records for business and tax reasons. Financial information should be systematically recorded, classified, summarized, and analyzed to promote effective business practices. There are four assumptions made. Business and personal finances will be kept separate. Next, the going concern states that the business will be around for a long time. Stable currency and business operations are recorded in timed increments. The four principles of accounting are: cost principle, revenue recognition, matching principle, and full disclosure. Cost Principle: acquisition costs are used not fair market values; Revenue Recognition: revenue is recorded when it is earned, not when received; costs are charged as expenses only when there is no connection between the cost and generated revenue; Matching Principle: expenses are matched with revenues; Full Disclosure: gathering information costs money so disclose only the necessary information.

Important terms

ABC Method: A type of classification for inventory which is done in accordance with the highest price to the lowest cost.

Account Balance: Debits that are subtracted from the credits to create this total or balance.

Account Payable: Purchases made on credit and the promise to pay in a timely manner.

Account Receivable: Payment promise from a customer for merchandise or service.

Account: A financial tool used to record increases or decreases in a business tally.

Accountant: Person whose job is the recording of financial data and the interpretation of the results based on the generated reports.

Accounting Cycle: Adjustments in between the recordings of a transaction and includes this process: Transaction => Documentation => Journal => Ledger => Trial Balance => Financial Statement. Each recording which happens within a specific time frame is called a fiscal period.

Accounting Equation: When the assets equal the liabilities plus the owner's equity.

Accounts Receivable Turnover: Average collection period for receivables and a computation derived by dividing net sales (or net credit sales) by average accounts receivable.

Accrual Accounting: Method where the expenses and revenues are recorded whether or not they are paid or received by the business.

Accrued Expense: Cost that is incurred but may not be paid by the business.

Accrued Income: this refers to revenue which is earned but may not be received by the business.

Acid Test Ratio: Quick ratio or a ratio which is inclusive of all the cash, cash receivables, notes receivables and accounts receivables that are summed then divided by the current liabilities.

Activity Analysis: Measure of effective use of assets within a business.

Actuating: The guidance and direction of the activities of a business or company.

Adjusted Trial Balance: Balance left after all entries have been adjusted and recorded.

Advertising: The company's marketing strategy to sell its wares or services.

Aftercare: The act of providing services after the initial need has been met as in the counseling services offered to a grieving family.

Age Discrimination in Employment Act of 1967: The legislation of Congress which states that all businesses are to treat all persons employed the same way regardless of their age.

Age of Accounts Receivable: Calculation derived by dividing 360 days by the receivable turnover time. The result is the measured time it takes to collect a receivable.

Aging Schedule: The accounting process which groups accounts according to the length of time payment has not been received.

Allowance for Doubtful Accounts: Uncollectible receivables which are bad debts.

Analyzing: Process of studying the financials of a business so that intelligent decisions can be made for the business.

Angels: The investors who provide start-up capital for small and/or risky business ventures.

Application Software: this term is given to programs loaded onto a computer to perform specified actions such as calculations, or compiling text in a word processing software. The software bridges the gap of the computer language of the computer into the language understood by humans.

Arithmetic Logic Unit: this is also known as ALU and is the part of the computer within the processing unit that calculates and solves logical problems.

Articles of Partnership: Title given to the document which outlines all obligations and commitments made by each person who has ownership investment within a specific business.

ASCII: this is the abbreviation for American Standard Code Information Interchange and it is a computer language code used for data.

Assembly Language: this refers to the converted language that is changed to a machine language within the Central Processing Unit and this conversion includes the grouped alphabet characters called mnemonics which replace number language.

Assets: Property with a monetary value owned by the business.

Average Collection Period: The amount of time it takes for the receivables or accounts to be collected.

Backup: this term refers to the duplication of data usually on an outside storage disk to guard against damage or loss in case of a computer crash or some other loss.

Balance Sheet: Formal financial statement that gives a complete overview of the fiscal situation of a company including all assets and all liabilities for a specific date of time.

Bank Draft: Order from an individual to a financial institution for withdrawal of a specific amount of monies to be paid to the bearer of the order.

Bank Statement Reconciliation: Procedure where an individual makes an assessment at the end of each month to determine the exact amount held in an account. All of the deposits and all the debits are balanced for a total and then the individual subtracts all checks written that are not included on the statement to determine the exact amount left in the account.

Bank Statement: this term refers to the financial document issued by a financial institution to inform an account holder of all activity on that account for a certain period of time.

Banker's Method: this is also known as the 360 day method which is a way to calculate interest based on a year comprised of 360 days.

Better Business Bureau: Private non-profit organization which has a membership of businesses that function as one service. The service maintains a data base on member businesses made available to the public concerning the number of complaints filed and/or settled by each business.

Bit: this term refers to the tiniest amount of information a computer can use.

Bona Fide Occupational Qualification: The compulsory requirements of a job as one discriminatory factor allowed by law.

Book Value: Cost of an asset minus its wear and tear and salvage value or depreciation.

Bookkeeper: this is also known as the Information Processor or the individual whose job is to record financial activity of a company.

Bookkeeping: Responsibilities of the bookkeeper in keeping the financial activity recordings of a company up to date.

Brand: Identification or name given to a certain product on the market.

Break-Even Analysis: Point when costs equal the income made from the sale of a service or product.

Budget: The formal document which outlines the coming year's reasonable expenditures and limiting of expenditures as based on previous years.

Burglary: Criminal act where forced entry is used to take or steal the moveable property and cash belonging to another person.

Business Interruption Insurance: Type of coverage that protects an owner from losses of income and/or property which are the result of a stated hazard on the policy such as a flood.

Business Plan: Title given to the document which has a description of a new venture. The project, marketing, budget, operating start-up capital, inventory, and all foreseeable events associated with the new business.

Business Policies: Term given to the management guidelines used in the day-to-day business affairs of a company.

Byte: this term refers to a single character space on a computer and is comprised of 8 bits of data.

Calendar Year: The 12 month period from January to December.

Cancelled Check: Document that indicates a paid financial order was returned to the original writer of the document.

Capital: Financial equity in a company or business.

Cash Accounting: Method that counts income earned when it is received and expenses are counted when they are paid.

Cash Basis Accounting: Method of accounting which counts receivables at the time the money comes in and not when the obligation happens.

Cash Disbursements: Cash payments or the legal tender or currency paid to a business.

Cash Discount: Markdown or reduction in price used as an incentive for prompt payment by a customer.

Cash Receipts Journal: Ledger where cash proceeds are recorded for a business.

Cash Short and Over: Ledger which traces inexplicable shortages or overages in cash as a perusal of the business transactions done.

Cash: All the liquid assets, currency, coin, credit cards, and/or money orders on hand.

Cashier's Check: A financial order drawn on a bank's own funds signed by an officer of the bank.

Casualty Insurance: Title given to the coverage that provides money to a business who has suffered a peril or hazard.

Cathode Ray Tube: this is also known as a CRT or a TV like contraption which when connected to a computer illustrates information via an electron beam which is controlled by the computer's phosphorescent screen.

Caveat Venditor: Refers to the phrase, "seller beware", used to indicate that a sale may not be all that it is portrayed to be due to some dishonest dealings by the buyer.

CD-ROM: this is the term given for an external storage disk which holds 700 megabytes of data or audio information. CD-ROM is short for Compact Disk-Read Only Memory.

Census of Business: Marketing data listing numbers and demographics of business enterprises.

Census of Housing: Data collected listing the demographics of residential domiciles within an area.

Census of Manufacture: this refers to the data collected listing the demographics of manufacturing businesses.

Census of Population: Data collected listing the demographics of a population in general in accordance with a specific region, state, county, or city.

Central Processing Unit: this is also known as the CPU and is the controlling part of the computer which obeys the instructions sent by the software. The CPU has three parts: primary storage (memory), arithmetic/logic unit, and the control unit.

Certified Check: A financial order guaranteed by the bank that the money is available to the holder of the check.

Certified Public Accountant: Abbreviated as C.P.A which is a licensed professional who has passed an exam of qualifying that person to work on the financial and tax matters of their clients.

Chain of Command: this refers to the rank of authority from superior to subordinate which determines who should be obeyed first. For example, a general's orders outrank a sergeant's orders.

Chamber of Commerce: Title given to the organization of businesses within a city or region which serves to create a more beneficial environment for the economic success of businesses in the area.

Chart of Accounts: Document that outlines all accounts and the numbers assigned to them in a specific format.

Check Stub: Record which illustrates what account the check was issued to for payment on that account.

Check: A financial order drawn upon an individual's account in a bank or financial establishment.

Chronological: Rank or order according to time.

Circulating Capital: Liquid assets of a company. The inventory and account receivables can also be included.

Civil Rights Act of 1964: Legislature which prevents discrimination to persons because of race, creed, religion, sex or national origin.

Classifying: Orderly arrangement and record of business transactions.

Closing Entries: Journal entries designed to empty the temporary accounts at the end of an accounting period for the transference to permanent accounts. This creates a summarization of the revenues and expenses for a specific period of time.

Coinsurance Clause: Provision which states that the insured must maintain an agreed upon percentage of the total value of property insured. One example of this is the 80/20 percentages where the owner maintains 80% of his insurance coverage and is liable for the 20% if a loss occurs.

Combination Journal: Original entry journal which encompasses the features of a two-column journal and a special journal in the ledger.

Competition: Business which strives to gain the business opportunities ahead of other like businesses. This can promote a healthy economy.

Compound Journal Entry: Recording of more than two accounts in the ledger.

Computer System: this term refers to the hardware and software working together for data processing purposes.

Computer: this term is given to a machine which controls information according to instructions through a series of components which work together to store data, retrieve data, change data, and release data according to instructions given to it.

Consumer Credit: Process individuals use for buying now and paying the loan off at a later date on an unsecured basis.

Consumerism: Protected rights of the consumer. This allows a safer, more trustworthy product to be purchased from the vendor.

Contra Account: Accumulated totals to counterbalance a related account.

Control Unit: this term refers to the part of the CPU which directs the sequence of operations, interprets the code into commands, and initiates commands to carry out the instructions for the computer.

Copyright: Legal registration showing that the written or created work is owned by the creator or the beneficiaries of the work produced.

Corporate Refugees: People who flee or leave big business settings within corporate America to start their own businesses.

Corporation Charter: State approved incorporation of a business in accordance to the written request of that business.

Credit Balance: Happens when the total of all credits in an account are greater than all the debits of the account in the given time frame.

Credit Bureau: Organization that keeps track of credit histories of individuals through the use of a summarized report of the businesses and organizations in which the individual has had dealings.

Credit Insurance: Protection given to a non-retail type of business who sustains losses due to non payments of the credit given to a customer.

Credit Memorandum: Source document which gives a buyer credit for purchase returned to the business.

Credit: Abbreviated as "CR" and always appears on the right side of an account.

Credit: Short term loan of money to buy something typically without the benefit of a security deposit or collateral.

Creditor: this refers to the individual or entity who grants credit to another person.

Cross Referencing: Procedure of entering transaction pages in the ledger and the journal in order to obtain the account number notation for that transaction.

Current Asset Ratio: Liabilities divided into assets currently existing within the business.

Current Assets: One year duration of cash or other asset consumption as it pertains to the operation of the business.

Current Liabilities: One year duration of liability's existence which is paid off in a year.

Current Ratio: Measurement of a business's liquidity by dividing assets by liabilities.

Customized Software: this term refers to a special set of instructions called a program which is designed to do a specific job for the user.

Data Input: this term refers to the information process which is entered into the computer by a data entry clerk.

Data Processing: this term refers to what the computer does with the information which results in reception, retrieval, duplication, and the production of information for use.

Data: this is the computer terminology which means information.

Database: this term refers to the information gathered into one place separated into specific categories or subjects.

Debit Balance: Total debits that amount to more than total credits in a ledger.

Debit: this term refers to the numbers which are always listed on the left side of an account ledger.

Debt Equity: Debt capital, borrowed capital, and any other capital which must be paid back.

Debtor: Individual or entity who owes a debt to a business.

Deductible Clause: Provision in insurance which makes the insured liable for the agreed upon deductible for a sustained loss of a thing which was insured.

Delegation of Authority: When a manager or superior gives the right for acting on the foundation's behalf over to someone else.

Demographics: Studies and gathered statistics on populations according to regions, income, density, preferences, and composition of families or businesses within a particular area.

Deposit Ticket: A deposit slip or a receipt of money deposited to an account in a financial institution.

Deposits in Transit: Monies made to an account which are not yet listed on the bank statement.

Depreciated Costs: A company's assets minus any liabilities and intangible assets listed in the ledgers of a company.

Depreciation Expense: Portion of the original cost of an asset which is recorded each year until the original cost is zeroed out on the books.

Depreciation: The financial consideration noting the wear and tear and salvage value of an asset held by a business.

Desktop Publishing: this term refers to the process of producing typeset printed material with a professional look or appearance.

Disaster: Any emergency, disaster, or catastrophe that results in loss of life, limb or property.

Disbursement: Payment of monies.

Discount Period: Amount of time a markdown is available for sale.

Dishonored Check: Financial order not paid by the bank which usually indicates that the funds are not available for withdrawal.

Disk: this term refers to the magnetic material which records bits of information for later retrieval or for storage backup use.

Display: this term refers to the visual information displayed on the computer screen or monitor.

Double Entry Accounting: Bookkeeping method whereby equal number of debits and credits are recorded for one transaction recorded.

Drawing Account: Owner withdrawal or when an equity account separate from the business equity account is drawn off for the owner's personal usage.

E.O.M.: Abbreviation indicating the end of the month.

Earnings Approach: Assessment of the value or worth of a business based on potential income.

Economic Base: Regionally based wealth or prosperity assessment which describes the jobs being performed within an area.

Economic Order Quantity: Point or position reached when total cost is at a minimum for the quantity purchased.

Endowment Life Insurance: Type of coverage which gives the insured the money in payment or lump sum according to face value when it matures.

Entrepreneur: A person who starts a business venture by himself.

Equal Employment Opportunity: Actions of employers in not practicing discrimination of people based on race, creed, religion, sex or nationality.

Evaluating: Controlling or managing methods which allows standards to be set that are used in comparison of job performance on an organizational and individual job performance level.

Expense: Efforts made to produce revenues that result in a decrease in asset or a withdrawal from an account.

Face of Note: The total an individual commits to pay in a loan or note.

Facilities Management: Maintenance of a work environment and the tools used in that environment.

Factoring: Act of selling customer accounts before they are paid in order to get cash now.

Federal Income Tax Withholding: Funds an employer pays to the government on behalf of the employee which are considered part of the employee's gross pay.

Federal Insurance Contributions Act: Abbreviated as F.I.C.A or the support of the federal social security program through payroll deduction.

Final Processing: Reporting method of summarizing all results accomplished during a fiscal period within a business operation.

Finance: Acquisition and utilization of money within a business or company.

Financial Management: Act of making use of the cash flow, assets, liabilities, and capital rights in a responsible manner to promote the success of a business.

Fiscal Period: The timeframe of an income statement generated for the business.

Fixed Assets: Also known as long term assets or property that is useful for a long time and not intended for resale.

Fixed Capital: All that is not cash: land, equipment, building, fixtures, and vehicles which are used as investments in small business enterprises.

Fixed Expenses: All liabilities which are set and cannot be changed due to any increase or decrease within the operation of the business. For example, the mortgage on a property is considered a fixed expense.

Fixed Liabilities: Also known as long term liabilities or notes or obligations that are not due within one year.

Floppy Disk: this term refers to a diskette or a small magnetic material which stores information for later use.

Follow-Up Services/Post-Need Service: Service offered by a funeral home which gives support to the bereaved after the final disposition has been rendered.

Footing: this is also known as the pencil footing or the total of a column of figures written in pencil at the bottom of a ledger.

Format: this term refers to the process which prepares a disk for information storage according to the computer's use requirements.

Funeral Service Management: Organization of the day-to-day business activities of a funeral home such as marketing, office administration, employee supervision, facility maintenance, and the like.

General Journal: this is also known as the original entry book where transactions are recorded according to chronological time.

General Liability Insurance: Type of coverage which protects the insured from unexpected injuries that customers may receive from an unexpected mishap or from products sold to the customer.

Gigabyte: this refers to the 1000 megabytes of information.

Goals/Objectives: An outline describing the business vision and the extent to which that business plans on achieving those aspirations.

Goodwill: Excellent reputation earned by the funeral home which enables it to earn a higher rate of profit than other funeral homes. This is an intangible asset of the business.

Graphics: this refers to the pictures or charts generated by the computer software.

Gross Earnings: this is also known as gross pay or the total income without deductions or taxes withheld from the entire amount.

Gross Profit Percentage: this term refers to the profit divided by sales in the form of a mathematical percentage.

Gross Profit: this is also known as the gross margin or the total of net sales with expenses of sales deducted already.

Hard Disk: this term refers to the fixed disk or the memory storage compartments found within the computer. This storage is read/write capable.

Hardware: this refers to the physical equipment, housing for the computer, disks, motherboard, and electronic cards that have instructions built in.

High-Level Language: this refers to the programming language which uses more than one machine language such as: BASIC, PASCAL, or COBOL.

Human Relations: Encouraging motivation which helps employees to develop teamwork, increase morale, and ultimately allows the company to achieve its goals.

Human Resource Forecast: The way business personnel needs are discovered and reported upon.

Human Resource Planning: The way in which a strategic preparation for future personnel needs is to be incorporated.

I/O: this refers to the abbreviation for Input/Output.

Immigration Reform Act: Regulation which requires all businesses to confirm the legality of a person working in the United States of America.

Impact Printer: this refers to the peripheral which prints characters by hitting the page with the ink-filled ribbon between the impact tool and the paper.

In Balance: this refers to the occurrence of having the debits and credits even out in the ledger.

Income statement: Profit and loss statement in past years. It is used to report a company's earnings over a specific period, usually a year. Income statements allow the owner to see how expenses are being controlled, taxes paid, interest accrued, and the rate of return a company is earning for the shareholders along with profit margins.

Income Statement: this is also known as a profit and loss statement or a statement of operations that works as the day to day operating summary of all revenues and sales from product and services including the amounts of profit or loss and all expenses incurred by the business.

Income: this is also referred to as revenue or all sales and revenue produced from sales of product or services from a business.

Independent Contractor: this term refers to an individual or company who agrees to do work for a fee without being under the control or the protection of the originating service providers.

Innovation: Modernization and upgrades given to allow for a new method or product to be put into use.

Input Device: this refers to the mechanized piece used to enter information into the computer.

Input: this refers to the information which is entered into the computer.

Installment Credit: Method of payment which allows a monthly payment of costly merchandise to be paid for over time.

Insurance: Coverage of any unexpected loss of monetary gain that could prove to be detrimental to the healthy flow of business. Such losses included things like fire, flood, and personal injury.

Intangible Asset: Anything which cannot be seen, held or put in the bank like a good reputation that gives confidence and credibility to a business which in turn adds to the business value.

Integrated Software: this refers to the programs which work together to allow information to be transferred from one application to another.

Interdependence: Dependence upon other business in a supportive relationship that helps each business be more productive and successful.

Interest: this term refers to the charge that is put on a sum of money for the use of that money in a transaction or loan.

Interpreting: this term refers to analyzing and comparing events then explaining them to others.

Interviewing: Act of asking questions and receiving answers. It is also a job study technique which explores a position by asking questions of a person who holds the desired position for a person looking to gain employment.

Inter-vivos: The trust which was set up by the deceased during his or her lifetime to ensure that property is held for a beneficiary as a gift with no compensation.

Inventory Turnover: Act of counting and categorizing the merchandise a company has on hand at the time of sale.

Inventory: this term refers to the documentation and the counting of items to be sold including the total amount of a purchase and the terms of payment for each item.

Job Analysis: Act of examining a position's critical factors in order to determine the skills required to do the work in a proficient manner.

Job Description: this refers to the list of duties required by a particular position in order to get the required work done in a proficient or acceptable manner.

Journal: this term refers to the book in which chronological entries of financial transactions for a company is kept.

Journalizing: Recording of transactions with date and explanations and amounts to be debited and credited and numbers of accounts affected by the transaction.

Key-Person Life Insurance: Coverage of loss should a particular person who is crucial to the efficient running of a business die.

Kilobyte: this is abbreviated as K/KB and is a measure of storage volume equal to 1024 bytes storage.

Language: this refers to the collection of characters which make sense as instructions to the computer.

Ledger: System of recording a group of accounts with the left side being the assets and the right side being the liabilities either in electronic forms or paperback forms.

Liabilities: this term refers to the debts owed by a company.

Liability Insurance: Coverage of loss resulting from any injury of a customer, or others, on premises or by product sold.

Line of Credit: Amount of available cash that can be borrowed from a bank based on the worthiness of a borrower to pay that amount back.

Liquidation Value: Amount which a business would be worth if everything owned by the business were sold.

Liquidity Analysis: this term refers to the evaluation of a company's ability to meet its financial obligations.

Local Area Network: this is abbreviated as LAN and occurs when several computers are linked in order to share peripherals such as printers.

Machine Language: this refers to the basic instructions written simply for the computer.

Mainframe: this refers to the central, controlling computer within a medium or large complex of computer systems.

Maker: this term refers to the individual who promises to pay or who signs a note of promise.

Management: The persons in charge and how they maintain that business, the employment motivations used, and the methods incorporated to run the business at optimum levels.

Manufacturing: Act of putting together raw materials into items that can be sold.

Markdown: Act of reducing a price on an item below suggested retail price for a quick sale.

Market Survey: Method used to discover the demographics that relate to what the potential customer "looks like" and where they are and what they want to buy.

Market Value Approach: Method used which establishes the worth or value of a business based upon the worth of similar businesses in the market place.

Market: Group of people that have the potential and desire to purchase that which is offered for sale.

Marketing: Act of advertising and packaging an item in such a way as to make people want to buy the product, good, or service that is for sale.

Markup: Act of raising the price of an item to allow a margin for profits to be earned by the company.

Maturity Date: this term refers to the day which a note comes due for payment.

Megabyte: this refers to the measurement of memory storage which equals 1, 048, 576 bytes of storage.

Memory Unit: this term refers to the place where the programs (software) and data are stored for usage at a later time.

Merchandise: this term is referred to as inventory or the goods which are intended for resale for profit from a sale.

Merchandising: Act of preparing finished goods for resale purposes.

Microcomputer: this refers to a desk top computer designed for personal use called a PC.

Modem: this refers to the computer's connection to a phone line through a device which converts electric, digital information into sound waves to send and receive input from the internet or from fax machines.

Monitor: this refers to the display screen which alerts the user to what the computer is doing with the input of data received from the user.

Mortgage Loan: Property-secured loan used for the purchase of property by a borrower.

Mortgage Payable: this term refers to a signed, written promise which uses real estate as a security for the payment from a liability which is long term due to the high cost of the property being purchased.

Mortgage: this refers to the amount of the payment or credit given to a borrower by the lender against property of the borrower.

Mouse: this refers to the device which moves a cursor over the screen in a point and click movement designed for interaction with the computer.

N.S.F.: this term refers to non-sufficient funds to cover a check presented to the financial institute.

Net Income: this term is also known as the net profit that occurs when gross profit is higher than expenditures going out.

Net Loss: this occurs when expenditures are higher than profits coming into the business.

Net Pay: this term refers to the net earnings or the amount on an employee's check which is gross pay minus all deductions.

Net Purchases: this term refers to the allowances with discounts deducted and purchases with returns deducted from the transaction.

Net Sales: this occurs when all returns and discounts are deducted from total sales for the period.

Network: this refers to a complex of computers hooked together electronically or wirelessly for the purpose of sharing peripherals and information with each other.

Non-Impact Printer: this refers to a peripheral which imprints paper with information without hitting the paper directly.

Note Payable: this term refers to a certain amount committed to be paid within a certain time frame.

Note Receivable: this term refers to a certain amount credited and paid within a certain time frame.

Occupational Safety and Health Act: Federal mandate directed towards employers to maintain a healthy and hazard-free environment for its employees.

Office Management: Supervision of the facility and functions of the business office within a company.

Open End Credit: Line of credit that can be used repeatedly until the monetary limit has been reached by the consumer.

Operating Expenses: this term refers to the overhead or expenditures that occur during day to day company functions in a business enterprise.

Operating Ratios: Income statement's percentage of sales which has derived income from the cost of items in comparison with profit margins set by the industry standards.

Operating System: this term refers to the set of instructions which helps the computer organize data into the applications for efficient use.

Organizing: Act of arranging the work flow in a systematic manner.

Original Cost Basis: this term refers to the amount paid for an asset which can be depreciated on the tax documents.

Other Expenses: this term refers to the expenditures which are made and are not a direct result of revenue production.

Other Income: this term refers to the revenue which results from activities other than normal sales and service of a company in a business enterprise.

Output: this occurs when the computer is finished processing a task and the data is sent to an output device such as the computer screen or the printer.

Outstanding Checks: this term refers to the commercial paper that has yet to be presented to the bank for payment which has already been given in payment of a purchase or service.

Overdraft: this occurs when a check is written without funds to cover the amount when it is presented for payment at the financial institution.

Overhead: Expenses accrued in the of running a business

Owner's Equity: this is also known as the net worth, or capital of a proprietorship's investment in the company which is figured by totaling the assets and subtracting the total liabilities of a company.

Partnership: Legal business arrangement where there are two or more owners of a business.

Patent: Registration of a product or invention by the owner or inventor. This also gives the owner the right to gain profit from the sale of the product or invention.

Payee: this term refers to the individual who receives the payment.

Peripherals: this refers to the input or output devices such as printer, mouse, or keyboard.

Personal Capital: Cash and/or assets of an individual which is invested in his or her own business venture.

Personnel Management: The organizing of employees into a workable and motivated group that gives the company an efficient work flow that is productive.

Petty Cash Fund: this term refers to the currency and coin set aside for small expenditures that occur on a daily basis.

Petty Cash Voucher: this term refers to the recording of a deduction from petty cash used.

Planning: Act of organizing for future needs of the company.

Post-Closing Trial Balance: this term refers to a report which reflects the temporary accounts transfer to the permanent accounts which reflect an equal amount in the debits and credits columns. .

Postdated Check: this term refers to a financial paper which is for a future payment on an account.

Posting to the ledger: Documenting of the two accounts that are affected by a transaction. A post of a credit and a debit must be made for every transaction.

Posting: this term refers to the recording from journal to the ledger.

Pre-Packaged: this term is also known as horizontal market software or off the shelf programs for general use by the consumer.

Prepaid Expenses: this term refers to the purchased assets that once used become expenses.

Primary: this is also known as internal storage or built-in memory used by the computer system.

Principal: this term refers to the face value of a note or loan to which interest will be added for the pay off amounts.

Printer: this is a term used to refer to a peripheral which imprints paper or similar material with data from a computer.

Processing: this is a term used for manipulating data within the computer system.

Product Liability Insurance: Coverage of loss derived from any injury from products sold.

Profit Margin: this term is derived by dividing the net income by the net sales in a transaction.

Profitability Analysis: this term refers to a report that illustrates effective management by showing the earning potential of a company.

Program: this is a term used to refer to the instructions in an application which tells the computer what to do with data that it has.

Programming: this is a term used to refer to the writing codes or the written instructions in a computer language which will tell the computer how to manipulate specific information efficiently.

Proving Cash: this term refers to the practice of determining that the total cash on hand and in the bank is equivalent to the final balance on the books.

Proving the Journal: this term refers to a page by page analysis used to confirm that the debits equal the credits.

Purchase Invoice: this term refers to the document which reflects items shipped, their cost and the shipment of the order.

Purchase Order: this term refers to the document which shows the authorization for buying a product or service in a transaction.

Purchase Requisition: this term refers to a document used to issue a request for buying an item or service. It is usually issued by the individual who does the buying in the company's stead.

Purchase: this term refers to the buying of a product or service in a transaction.

Purchases Discount: this term refers to contra temporary account where discounts are recorded due to a markdown on price from bulk buying or prompt payments.

Purchases Journal: this term refers to the book where buying on credit occurrences only are recorded in chronological order in the ledger.

Purchases Returns and Allowances: this term refers to a contra account where returns of defective items to the manufacturer are recorded by the bookkeeper.

Quarterly: this term refers to the parts of the year in one quarter increments or in 3 months increments.

Quick Assets: this term refers to receivables, cash, and securities that are marketable for sale.

Random Access Memory: this term is used to refer to the RAM or the working memory of the computer which holds applications for use and efficiently stores the data in the computer system.

Rate: this term refers to the percentage used to compute interest usually on an annual basis in a calculation.

Read-Only Memory: this is also known as ROM or storage which cannot be changed by the user because it is protected, pre-programmed memory used for the operation of the computer.

Recording: this is also known as data entry or the act of writing down financial events.

Recruitment: Gathering of applicants for the purpose of filling open positions in a company for employment needs.

Replacement Value Approach: Reasonable cost of restoring property or products after a loss.

Restrictive Endorsement: this occurs when an individual controls the use of commercial paper signed by the individual or controls what the paper will buy in a transaction.

Resume: Documentation listing a person's education and previous employment along with skills and job proficiency in an effort to obtain a position in a company.

Retail Sales Tax: this term refers to the tax imposed by state, county and municipalities on items sold by the business.

Risk Management: Financial method of reducing risk while preserving the assets and earning power of a business.

Salary: this term refers to the compensation for work done usually in a managerial capacity for a company.

Sales Discount: this refers to the contra account which records the discounts given to customers for prompt payment using a markdown to gain payment from the customers.

Sales Invoice: this term refers to the document which is given by the seller to the buyer outlining the particulars of a sale.

Sales Journal: this term refers to the records of chronological sales on a credit basis.

Sales Promotion: Advertising and marketing strategies used to gain sales.

Sales Returns and Allowances: this term refers to the contra account in which credits for the defective merchandise returns are recorded.

Sales: this refers to a temporary account set up to record revenue generated by exchange of product for money or services for money by the company.

Secondary: this is also known as external storage or the disk units outside the computer's main hard drive memory unit.

Self-Insurance: Process where an organization sets aside a portion of earnings to ensure that monies are available in case of a loss from worker's compensation, medical expenses, and/or a loss of properties.

Service Business: Company whose business is derived from a service rather than merchandise sold.

Small Business Administration: The SBA or governmental agency responsible for assisting small businesses in the acquisitions of government contracts. The SBA also gives loans for capital improvements to small businesses and helps in providing information about sound business practices.

Small Business: Company with less than 1500 employees that does not control or lead in its industry and has less than $13 million in annual sales.

Software: this term refers to an application which can be for general use such as word processing or for accounting purposes.

Source Document: this is also known as business paper or the first piece of paper recording a transaction such as receipts or invoices.

Special Journal: this term refers to a single type transaction recording by the bookkeeper.

Spreadsheet: this term refers to accounting ledgers within the computer which contain the capability to handle numeric calculations and to organize numeric data efficiently.

Staffing: The act of seeking, gaining, training, and evaluating employees.

Statement of Account: this term refers to a document prepared by the merchant which outlines the status of a customer's accounting transactions with the company.

Statement of Owner's Equity: this is also known as the statement of net worth or the document which proves the changes in the owner's equity during a specific time frame.

Statistical Program: this refers to specific software which handles statistical information to be retrieved by the user.

Stop Payment Order: this occurs when an individual requests that the bank not pay a check or commercial paper when presented for payment by the holder.

Storage Device: this refers to the unit which houses memory disks or tape units for backup purposes.

Store: this refers to the act of transmitting data to memory for storage.

Straight Line Depreciation: this term refers to the actual cost of an asset when divided into equal amounts and recorded as expense over the useful lifetime of the item recorded.

Summarizing: this term refers to the gathering of all financial information into reports or statements for the company principals in an effort to bring clarity to the financial status of the company.

Supercomputer: this refers to a larger and faster computer used mainly for huge jobs such as scientific or government work operations.

Supplies: this term refers to the items used to manufacture a product for the business enterprise.

T Account: this term refers to the arrangement of an account with title on top, debits on left side and credits on the right side making the shape of a T on the page.

Tangible Asset: this term refers to an item which is of a physical form and has an absolute value of worth.

Temporary Owner's Equity Accounts: this term refers to accounts which denote income, expenses and withdrawals for a specified time frame.

Terabyte: this term refers to one thousand gigabytes of information used for computer storage.

Term Life Insurance: Protective coverage that comes without a cash value at the end of the policy when a loss is due to a death.

Time: this is also known as the term of the note or the period which the individual is given to pay for an item or service bought on credit by a consumer.

Total Quality Management: Tool which requires that all employees of an organization participate in the process of improving the production of product and in the problem solving of inefficiencies that occur within the work environment.

Trade Credit: Financial aid between businesses where one company gives credit to another so that product can be distributed.

Trademark: Logo or brand name which is registered and identifies a company.

Transaction Analysis: this is the term given for a study of business effects.

Transposition Error: this occurs when an amount is written with all the digits written correctly, but in the wrong order as the original number.

Trial Balance: Total that is gained from recording a transaction as follows: Transaction => documentation => Journal => Ledger => Trial Balance => Financial Statement.

Uncollectible Accounts: Bad debts expense or the loss from uncollectible accounts from the receivables which are not paid and prove to be uncollectible.

Universal Life Insurance: Type of coverage from a death loss that is combined with a whole life and term life policy.

Useful Life: this is the term that refers to the period of time an item can be utilized in business without becoming obsolete or worn out for use.

Utility Program: this term refers to software which manages the operation of the computer itself, not application software which manipulates the data used by the computer.

Variable Expense: Cost which stays constant or the same in regards to each unit of product. However, the total will go up or down in price depending upon total volume of the unit.

Venture Capitalist: Investor of a new business.

Vertical Market Software: this term refers to specific industry software which is not used by the general public.

W-2 Form: this is the title given for the Wage and Tax Statement provided to the Internal Revenue Service and to the employee that denotes gross earnings and all deductions including Medicare and Social Security taxes.

W-4 Form: this is the title given to the certificate that denotes an employee's withholdings.

Wage is denoted in an hourly or weekly amount as compensation for skilled or unskilled labor or for pieces done.

Word Processing: this term refers to the software which causes written documents to be produced by computerized equipment through data input by the user.

Worksheet: this is the term used for the spreadsheet which computes, sorts, and classifies accounts before the actual final financial statement is compiled for use.

Embalming

Formaldehyde spills

OSHA laws for formaldehyde spills require that small containers should be used in the cleanup process. The leaking container should be placed or situated in a well ventilated area to prevent harmful effects. Small spills can be cleaned with absorbent materials. The absorbent materials should be placed into a properly labeled container for disposal at a later time. You should dike a larger spill or in some way minimize contamination of the spill. Then facilitate the removal of the contaminated product from the workplace. You may be able to neutralize the spill with a solution of sodium hydroxide or sodium sulfite. EPA rules require employers to comply with regulations regarding clean-up of toxic waste. State and local authorities should be notified as required. Spills greater than 1,000 lb/day must be reported in accordance with EPA's Superfund legislation. Unofficial neutralization chemicals for small spills include the use of ammonia and kitty litter.

Protective clothing

OSHA has set guidelines regarding the protective clothing needed when using concentrations of formaldehyde greater than 1%. Negative pressure respirators with approved canisters or cartridges are restricted and are not allowed for use in a full work shift. Positive-pressure air purifiers or self-contained breathing apparatuses should be used to provide a measure of safety. Protective gloves are also recommended for use. The gloves should be selected to provide the least amount of permeation in accordance with the ACGIH guidelines. Goggles or some type of complete eye protection from splashes or sprays and a face shield are needed. However, one should not use the face shield alone as this does not provide adequate eye protection. Clothing should be impervious to permeation. The employer is responsible to provide the employee with a private chamber for changing, an emergency shower, and an eye wash fountain.

Chemical properties of formaldehyde

Methanal is the simplest aldehyde. Methanal has the chemical formula H_2CO. A structural formula $HCHO$ has a colorless gas with a definite pungent or strong smell. This chemical is dehydrating to mucous membranes. Dehydration refers to the removal of water from matter. This dehydration affects the skin to a lesser degree. It is readily soluble in water at a saturated level of 37%. At this saturated level it is called formalin. Silver, iron oxide, molybdenum, and vanadium act as catalysts to produce the oxidation processes needed for methanol. A polymer is a substance formed by bonding several monomers or basic chemical units through a process called polymerization. Once polymerized it dries to a state called paraformaldehyde. In basic solution it is unstable. In its basic solution it will decompose in an alkaline surrounding medium. It will polymerize if the medium becomes too acidic.

The basic solution will react with ammonia to form urotropin. Urotropin forms into a crystalline state or condition. The remains of a deceased body that is well on the way to decomposition and in advanced decomposition require much higher concentrations of formaldehyde. This occurs because of the fact that HCHO has an affinity or attraction for nitrogen. Nitrogen is a crucial element found in protein. When protein hydrolyzes, more nitrogen is out in the open. Hydrolyze refers to the action of water breaking down a compound to form an acid and a base composition. This causes the formaldehyde to react with the nitrogen. Other factors can cause this nitrogen and formaldehyde reaction. One example of this is found in uremic poisoning or blood found in the urine. Uremic poisoning can also cause this effect because urea has the nitrogen element.

Types of embalming fluids

The condition of the remains determines the strength, volume and type of fluid to be used. In the case of excess fluid in the abdomen, excess fluid must be drained so the cavity embalming fluid can properly preserve the area. In addition, this prevents purge from draining from the mouth or nose. Embalmers should also pack the anus with disinfectant-soaked cottons. Jaundiced or emaciated remains do require large volumes and higher concentrations of fluids. However, the embalmer must be cautious because astringent fluids can cause formaldehyde burn and tissue discoloration on the skin. In addition, the decedent may have a colostomy or gastronomy tube. All medical devices should be disinfected and deposited in hazardous medical waste disposal containers. Open wounds should be dried, disinfected, sutured and packed with absorbent material and covered with plastic to prevent leakage.

Cavity and arterial fluids

The purpose of cavity fluids is to preserve and de-germ the interior of the body cavity. For this reason, the cavity fluid will contain high concentrations of disinfectants and preservatives. The cavity fluids generally lack any treatments with dyes, deodorants or modifying agents as part of its solution. This is due to the fact that there is generally no need for cosmetic treatment to the thoracic and abdominal cavities and their organs found in the body. The composition of the cavity fluid will have a higher acidic pH (4.5 to 5.2) content. This high acidic content gives it an excellent reaction with the tissue proteins. Arterial fluids have dyes for aesthetic or cosmetic reasons. Deodorants were previously called reodorants. The deodorants are responsible for covering up the harsh chemical smells from the other treatments received by the body.

Surfactants help the flow and the diffusion of the embalming fluids. Surfactants are surface wetting agents and surface-tension reducing agents. Other arterial fluids include: modifying agents, germicides, preservatives, and anticoagulants. The preservatives used are aldehydes, alcohol, phenolic compounds, and germicides. Phenolic compounds are compounds that preserve and disinfect because they precipitate protein. Modifying agents are required in embalming fluids due to the caustic nature of disinfectants and preservatives which scorch delicate capillaries causing a fluid diffusion problem. They delay the actions of the disinfectants and preservatives until adequate fluid has been soaked up by the tissues. The EDTA recommends certain agents to dilute the ionized calcium blood clotting effects, the chelates, and the calcium ions in the blood. Sodium citrate does the same thing; however sodium citrate will react with certain bacterial enzymes and coagulate the blood.

Preservatives and modifying agents

The preservatives used in embalming fluids are aldehydes, alcohols, phenolic compounds, and germicides. Aldehydes are cross link proteins. One of the most common forms of preservatives is known as formaldehyde. Formaldehyde is a lower aldehyde and provides many more cross links for more tissue firmness and provides a barrier to decomposition. Alcohol such as methanol, ethanol and isopropyl alcohol are sometimes used in conjunction with aldehyde in the embalming process. Methanol is used more often because of the dual properties of preservative and because it is an antipolymerizing agent. Ethanol and isopropyl are germicides. However, isopropyl is less costly than ethanol. Phenolic compounds are compounds that preserve and disinfect. These qualities are due to the phenolic compounds ability to precipitate protein. Phenols are used as bleaching agents. Phenols can create a putty-gray color when used with aldehydes in the embalming process.

The preservative known as quaternary ammonium is used as a surface disinfectant. Another preservative known as glutaraldehyde has been labeled the "cold chemical sterilant". Modifying agents are required in embalming fluids due to the caustic nature of disinfectants and preservatives. This caustic nature can scorch delicate capillaries and cause a fluid diffusion problem. They delay the actions of the disinfectants and preservatives until adequate fluid has been soaked up by the tissues. Humectants help the tissues retain moisture so they are not dried out by the aldehydes and alcohols. Humectants are glycols, glycerols, sorbitols, other polyhydroxy alcohols, and soluble lanolin compounds. Buffers are stabilizers which resist any changes in pH. Formaldehyde polymerizes in acidic conditions and decomposes in alkaline conditions. Examples are borax, sodium phosphate, citrates and sodium salts. Methyl Alcohol is routinely added to arterial fluids to combat polymerization of formaldehyde.

Embalming methods for infants

Embalming methods on infants require caution. The femoral and carotid arterial incisions should be avoided due to problems associated with pressure, flow rate, and the fluid index or coloration. A much better distribution is given when the thoracic incision is considered. In this incision the embalmer should remove part of the sternum. Partial extraction of the heart from the pericardial sac is followed by the insertion of a tube into the left ventricle using a small incision in the right ventricle for drainage. The pumping station is used at a pressure of 1 to 1.5 pounds on a slow rate to avoid swelling. Aspirate through the incision, then add 6 to 12 oz of cavity fluid. Place the heart back into the thoracic cavity, replace the sternum, suture the opening, and apply a light coating of sealant or adhesive bandage to keep any fluids from leaking from the site.

Bone and joint disorders

An experience funeral director will be aware of the skill required in the restorations which involve fractures. Facial swelling or cranial swelling can occur when a skull fracture is not noticed by the embalmer. Head freeze is a technique in which both carotids are cannulated and perfused at high pressure at the same time in an attempt to avoid distortions. This also preserves the brain and gives the facial features a plump and full look. Arthritic joints are misshapen and swollen and the edema is extravascular. Surface embalming may be required. However, rearrangement of the joints or bone structure may require written permission from the next of kin. Bone procurement means that the decedent has donated bone. This requires specialized embalming procedures because the bones are removed from the leg, hip, feet, and arm.

Governing governmental agencies

Each state in the United States regulates the embalming process according to legislative acts. Generally, one or two boards will have control over the dead body: the board of health and/or a state board of funeral directors and embalmers. There are other entities which will come into play during the embalming process to ensure the safe and legal disposition of the deceased. These include the Environmental Protection Agency (EPA), the Centers for Disease Control (CDC), the Federal Trade Commission (FTC), and the Occupational Safety and Health Administration (OSHA) along with various state agencies.

Importance of historical Egypt

It is generally considered that Egypt is where embalming first began considering their long history for mummification. It is thought that Egyptians developed embalming for two prime reasons: religion and sanitation. The Egyptians believed that the soul was immortal and as long as the body remained intact the soul would never forsake the body. Embalming was the method for the soul to complete what was called the circle of necessity which was a 3,000 mile journey the soul took before it was allowed to return to reunite with the body. The reunited soul and body could then rise up as a whole man and live with the gods. In addition, embalming was a measure used to counteract the tendency of the Nile River to flood which would bring to the surface buried bodies and cause further deaths due to the presence of the dead bodies.

Reasons for embalming

Embalming is performed for three reasons. The first is to disinfect the deceased. Dangerous pathogenic organisms can survive for long periods of time in dead tissues. Since most bodies are not buried immediately, there is the potential for spread of disease from those coming in contact with the deceased or for the spread of disease through insects which may land on the body. Another purpose for embalming is to preserve the body prior to viewing and burial. Decomposition and putrefaction begins soon in the deceased and this preservation process will slow down these factors and lessen odors. The third purpose is to restore the body to a more life-like appearance for the viewing portions of the memorial service and funeral.

Embalming process steps

The embalming process begins with the removal of clothing and any accessories. The body is then placed face up on the embalming table, washed and disinfected. The face will be shaved if the deceased is normally clean-shaven. The eyes will be closed by use of an eye cap under the eyelid. The mouth will be closed, the jaws fastened shut and the lips placed in a natural lip line, using glue if necessary. The embalming solution will be prepared prior to an incision being made over the carotid artery or the femoral artery and the artery and vein will be isolated. The artery and vein will be cannulated and embalming fluid will be injected into the artery under pressure and fluid will drain from the vein. The tubes are then removed and the incision is then sutured.

A trocar is used to tap the abdominal cavity to remove gases and fluid by suction and preservatives will be placed into the abdominal cavity. The body will then again be washed, the hair shampooed and finger nails cleaned. The face, hands and lips will be treated with cream to prevent dehydration. In final preparation, cosmetics will be applied to replace natural color lost due to blood loss; women will have their normal cosmetics applied. The hair will be combed or set in the style worn by the deceased. The body will then be dressed and placed into the casket.

Types of death

The following types of death:
- Necrobiosis: this is the death of cells over the lifespan of a living organism. The dead cells are replaced by living ones continuously over the lifespan of the organism.
- Necrosis: this is when many cells die in one particular organ or part of an organ.
- Clinical death: this happens immediately after brain activity, breathing and circulation ceases. There is a small possibility that this can be reversed if immediate life saving measures is taken.

- Brain death: this occurs when the brain is starved of oxygen for three to seven minutes. The brain will be the first organ to die if respiration or circulation ceases. After this happens the brain cannot be brought back to life.
- Somatic death: this is the death of the organism as a whole and generally occurs after brain death.

Ethical obligations

Some of the ethical considerations for embalmers are as follows. The embalmer is charged with judicious counseling for the deceased person's family members on funeral preparation. Other responsibilities the embalmer should take is to observe all regulations and rules pertaining to the handling of the deceased; properly identifying and handling the deceased; protect the health of the public through control and sanitation of the deceased; assisting the family to view their deceased family member or with organ donation requests; they should not misrepresent their credentials nor make derisive statements about other embalmers; and embalmers should maintain their credentials through further education and training.

Embalming methods

There are four primary methods used in embalming: cavity, hypodermic, surface and vascular. **Cavity embalming** consists of the direct treatment of using a trocar in the three body cavities-the abdominal, the pelvic and the thoracic. **Hypodermic embalming** is performed on tissues which cannot be treated via vascular embalming. A syringe and needle or a trocar is used. **Surface embalming** is done on the surface tissues through use of direct contact with chemicals used to preserve the body. **Vascular embalming** is the most common way to introduce embalming fluids into the body. The fluids are introduced into the body by use of the vascular system to disseminate the solutions to most parts of the body.

Embalming hazards

The embalmer will be presented with a number of hazardous conditions in the course of embalming. The chemicals used in the embalming process pose the greatest risk to the embalmer. Contact with these chemicals can cause dermatitis and eye, nose and lung irritations. Use of appropriate protective gear will help minimize these hazards but may also prove a hazard to the embalmer. They can trap body heat, increase personal humidity and be poorly ventilated. The deceased body can expose the embalmer to radiation (if the body was treated in this manner) and biological hazards such as infectious agents.

Hazard protection

The embalmer should always wear appropriate personal protective equipment (PPE) which will prevent infectious materials (blood, body fluids) from leaking through to the skin, mouth, eyes, nose and clothing. A rule of thumb is that no skin should be exposed. The PPE consists of gloves, head covering (cap, hood), face shield, eye goggles/safety glasses, long-sleeved protective body garment, and non-slip, water resistant foot coverings. The gloves should be thick latex or nitrile gloves. Regular latex gloves are not suitable. If the equipment is not disposable they should be appropriately cleaned and laundered. Disposable garments should be properly disposed in suitable containers.

Complicating illnesses

Renal failure will cause complications during the embalming procedure due to a number of changes to the body. There will be an increase in ammonia (which can neutralize formaldehyde) and fluid retention (edema). Uremia will cause pruritus of the skin and typically the skin will be a sallow color. Added complications to renal failure can be congestive heart failure, pulmonary edema and gastrointestinal bleeding. Liver failure can also cause an increase in ammonia, jaundice (yellowish discoloration to the skin), and hair loss. In addition to these complications liver failure can cause gastrointestinal bleeding, esophageal bleeding due to ruptured veins and excessive purges.

Algor mortis

There are a number of physical changes which occur postmortem. One change is algor mortis which is the cooling of the body after death. The body will start to cool until it reaches ambient room temperature. A number of factors will influence algor mortis: illness prior to death, infection, high room temperature, activity just prior to death, and decomposition. The Glaister equation can be used to determine the approximate time of death. It is 98.4% minus the measured rectal temperature of the body divided by 1.5. This gives the approximate hours since the death occurred.

Rigor mortis and liver mortis

Rigor mortis occurs gradually after death. It is the onset of rigidity to the body caused by the conversion of glycogen stores into lactic acid. The muscles are not shortened during this process. The excessive lactic acid causes a cross-linking of actin and myosin. Heat, acidosis, uremia and some other medical conditions which lower the pH of the body will accelerate the rate of rigor mortis. It will usually dissipate within 12 to 36 hours after death.

Liver mortis occurs when blood pools in the dependant areas of the body. Without the heart's pumping action the blood will seep into the lowest parts of the body and cause the capillary beds in these areas to expand with the blood. Usually the areas where the blood pools will be a purple or dark blue color. It reaches its maximum settling at eight to twelve hours after death.

Sequence of events

Death will usually follow a sequence of events. These include the **ante mortem period, agonal period**, and then **somatic death**.

The **ante mortem period** sets the stage for life to cease. The agonal period is the sequence of events that occurs just prior to death. Somatic death means all functions which sustain life have ceased and the body's cells are dead. The signs of death include the cessation of breathing, the cessation of circulation, muscles become flaccid, the eye exhibits changes such cornea cloudiness, the eyeball flattens, and the pupils become dilated. Postmortem lividity will then set in, followed by rigor mortis, then algor mortis and then eventually decomposition.

The **agonal period** is the ante mortem state right before death. It is the sequence of events that leads to the inability of the body to sustain metabolic and physiological activities which are necessary to sustain life. During the agonal period (pre-death changes) a number of things happen. There is a change in circulation where the blood thickens (agonal coagulation). Respiration and circulation slows causing agonal hypostasis. Coagulation causes agonal capillary expansion where the capillary walls swell then rupture due to the thickened blood. Blood serum escapes from the intravascular system to extravascular locations causing agonal edema. There will also be a loss of moisture and fluid to the environment eventually causing agonal dehydration.

Post mortem changes

Post mortem changes occur to the human body. These include algor mortis, liver mortis, dehydration, hypostasis, thickened blood, rigor mortis, post mortem stains, pH changes to the body and eventually decomposition. Decomposition will involve two major changes to the body tissues. One is autolysis which usually starts in the pancreas. Digestive enzymes in the cells will break down the proteins and carbohydrates. Autolysis is a minor component of decomposition. Putrefaction is the main component of decomposition. It is caused by bacterial activity which causes gas to form which in turn causes the body to bloat. Hydrogen sulfide gas will cause a brown-black discoloration in the blood vessels. The abdomen will take on a green discoloration. Finally the skin will blister and slip, and the nails and hair will be lost.

Effects of rigor mortis

Rigor mortis will affect the amount of fluid taken up by the tissues, and injection of fluid under high pressure during rigor mortis may cause tissue swelling. Tissue will take up embalming fluid at different rates. From lowest uptake to highest the tissue uptake of fluid will be arterial walls and skin, muscle and viscera. When rigor mortis sets in the blood vessels will contract and restrict the flow of the fluid to the tissues. When the body is in rigor mortis it will be difficult to sufficiently inject enough embalming fluids. If the body is embalmed at the start of rigor mortis, the embalmer may assume that enough fluids have been injected into the tissues when in fact rigor has set in. This will lead to lack of sufficient fluids to adequately preserve the body.

Important terms

Accessory Chemicals: these are a collection of chemicals (not including the embalming fluids used in the vascular system) which include hardening compounds, mold preventative agents, preservation powders, sealing agents, and pack application chemicals.

Aneurysm Hook: this is an embalming tool used to raise vessels and to perform blunt dissection. The hook end has an eye to aid in placing ligatures around the blood vessels.

Angular Spring Forceps: this is a versatile tool used during embalming.

Arterial Tube: this is a tube which is used when injecting embalming fluid into the blood vascular system.

Autoclave: this piece of equipment is used to sterilize items using steam and pressure.

Bridge Suture (Interrupted Suture): this type of tissue is used to align tissues using separate stitches which are knotted at the edge of the tissues.

Bulb Syringe: this soft rubber pump is used to manually create pressure in order to deliver fluid. The fluid passes through one way valves which are found in the bulb and it cannot be used to aspirate fluids.

Calvarium Clamp: this clamp is used to refasten the calvarium after a cranial autopsy has been performed.

Decay: Has two meanings. The first meaning is the decomposition of the proteins in a body by aerobic bacteria enzymes. The second meaning is the change of the body from a state of soundness due to the destructive dissolution of the body. This usually is a slow change over time.

Decomposition: The separation of complex compounds into less complex substances or simple elements due to the actions of microorganisms and enzymes.

Drain Tubes: these tubes are inserted into a vein as an aid to drainage of blood while restricting the exit of embalming fluid. They will be of varying sizes and diameters and will usually have a plunger.

Drench Shower: this OSHA required safety device is used to rinse a person off using large amounts of water. Used if a person has been contaminated with hazardous materials.

Electric Spatula: this is a heated blade (electric) which is used to dehydrate or reduce tissues and to restore contour to tissues.

Embalming: The process which uses chemicals on a dead body to sanitize and preserve the body. The chemicals used will slow decomposition and lower the number of microorganisms which decompose the body. During this process, the body's proteins are changed into new proteins which are more stable and do not retain water. Embalming is also used to restore the body to an acceptable appearance.

Eye Wash Station: this equipment is required by OSHA and is designed to flush the eyes using a stream of water.

Eyecap: this is a device used to help close the eyes. It is a plastic cup shaped disk inserted under the eyelids.

Gravity Injector: this device relies on gravity to deliver embalming fluid into the vascular system.

Groove Director: this tool is used when guiding vein tubes into the blood vessels.

Head Rest: this device is used during the embalming process to keep the head in an appropriate position.

Hydroaspirator: this device is connected to a water supply. When the water valve is opened, suction develops which allows the operator to aspirate the body cavity contents.

Mortuary Putty: this is a paste use to fix or fill defects.

Nasal Tube Aspirator: this tool is used during embalming to aspirate throat contents via the nostrils.

Needle Injector: this piece of equipment is used to place metal pins into bone.

Packing Forceps: this device is used to fill packing into the body's external orifices.

Personal Protective Equipment: this is clothing and equipment designed to protect the user from hazards.

Positioning Devices: these devices are used to position the body during the process of embalming.

Preparation Room: this is a room designated for embalming and for other preparations of the body.

Preservation: The methods used to treat the dead body with chemicals to prevent decay and to slow decomposition. However, given the proper temperature, humidity levels and environment, preservation can occur without chemical use.

Putrefaction: What occurs when organic matter is decomposed by anaerobic bacteria or by fungi which form foul-smelling products which are not completely oxidized.

Sanitation: Process which uses techniques which will establish conditions which stop biohazards.

Scalpel: this instrument, which has a handle and a removable disposable blade, is used to make incisions and excisions in the body during the embalming procedure.

Sterilizer: this is an oven or appliance, such as an autoclave, which is used to sterilize equipment. It will typically use steam under pressure to achieve sterility.

Trocar button: this device is made of plastic and has a threaded, screw-like shaft. It is used to seal punctures or the openings created in the body by the trocar.

Trocar: this is a sharp pointed tool which is used to aspirate body cavities and to inject the cavity with fluid. It may supplement hypodermic embalming.

Restorative Art

Overview

Restorative art involves the renovation of the human features to a state that is more pleasing and lifelike in appearance. The cause of death can have an impact on whether or not this process can be accomplished. In some cases, it may be necessary to refrain from this process. Some causes of death make the rearrangement of the facial features too difficult to allow a more natural form possible. The condition of the body may make this process difficult. The psychological benefit derived from viewing the body makes the effort of restoration a worthwhile endeavor. A Funeral Director's effort in producing these restorative results after an unnatural death can create an opportunity for an intangible asset. The intangible asset is the word of mouth advertising where a client expresses satisfaction. Facial restoration can be critical due to the fact that the face is viewed more often than other portions of the body.

Minor and extensive types

The most minor restorative art is found in the application of cosmetics, hair coiffeur, and setting of facial features into natural placement. Those closest to the decedent will be viewing the face. Therefore, setting the features of the face should be performed with care. Removal of skin blemishes, sub tissue surgery, bleaching, removing discolorations and rehydration of tissues may be necessary to create a more natural appearance. The family should be informed of the time involved and the complexity of the removal of a tumor, reduction of a tumor or swelling, repair of major fractures or breaks, removal of cancer areas and replacement of tissue, and the manipulation of deep wounds. Most of the restoration must be done after the arterial embalming. Some must be done before the embalming, due to the fact that corrective colorations are chemically achieved. The embalmer will require technical skill and some surgical skill.

Important terms

Abrasions: this term refers to the scrapes which cause skin to be removed after death has occurred.

Abscess: this term refers to the collection of pus in one area deep under the skin of the body.

Absorption: this term refers to the soaking up of certain rays of light or color so that the light is not reflected in a restorative art process. For example, black absorbs light and white reflects it.

Abut: this term refers to when one object is connected to another or comes up against the other.

Acetone: this term refers to a chemical known as dimethyl ketone which is a chemical liquid that has the ability to dissolve wax, remove stains, or soften and remove scabs.

Achromatic Color: this term refers to a neutral color such as white or black, gray or other decorative color that is not visible in light.

Acquired Facial Markings: this term refers to the wrinkles, lines, and grooves in the face caused by using certain facial muscles. Some examples are laugh lines or crow's feet at the eye corners.

Additive Method: this term refers to a process used in lighting where two colors of light are mixed to create another color.

Adhesive: this term refers to a sticky substance which causes two surfaces to stay together or adhere together.

After-Image: this occurs when the eye is stimulated by an object or light and then the stimulus is removed, but the object or light is still seen in a negative or a black and white form.

Airbrush: this term refers to an art form that atomizes the paint onto the surface with air.

Alveolar Process: this term refers to a bony ridge which holds the teeth sockets and projects from the inferior surface of the maxilla and superior surface of the mandible within the body.

Alveolar Prognathism: this term refers to the portion of the facial structure that juts out to hold the sockets for the teeth.

Amputate: this term refers to that which is cut off from the body.

Analogous: this term refers to colors that have similarities, but are different enough to highlight a contrast.

Anatomical Guide: this term refers to the descriptive guide which refers to the positions of arteries and veins by way of anatomical markers.

Anatomical Position: this term refers to the standing erect with feet and palms facing forward.

Anchor: this term refers to the technique which secures tissues or restorative substances in place.

Angle of the Mandible: this term refers to the junction of the lower jaw (the posterior edge of the ramus and the inferior surfaces of the mandible) that make an angle.

Angle of Projection: this term refers to the degree of protrusion an object or feature makes from the vertical surface.

Angulus Oris Eminence: this term refers to the small convex space at the end of the lips when closed.

Angulus Oris Sulcus: this term refers to the end of closed lips which makes a groove.

Antemortem: this term refers to the period after death.

Anterior: this term refers to the ventral or abdominal side of the body.

Anterior Nares: this term refers to the openings of the nostrils in the face.

Antihelix: this term refers to the ear's inner rim.

Antitragus: this term refers to the projection or the bulge opposite the tragus, bounding the cavum conchae posteroinferiorly and continuous above the anthelix.

Aqueous: this term refers to the water-filled or water-downed condition of something.

Aqueous Humor: this term refers to the thin, alkaline fluid that fills the eyeball.

Aquiline: this term refers to a hooked–nose or beak-like shape to the nose.

Arch: this term refers to a structural shape that is curved upward similar to a taut bow or curve.

Areolar: this term refers to the tissue within the body that connects things and fills spaces of the body.

Armature: this term refers to the frame used by the restorative artist in a wax restoration.

Aspiration: this term refers to the action which causes the removal of liquid or gases by suction.

Asymmetry: this term refers to the sides that are similar but not exactly identical on both sides of a thing.

Bandage: this term refers to a wrapping of material or cotton or gauze which is secured around a wound or injury.

Base: this term refers to a cosmetic which is used to make the face a standard color.

Basic Pigment: this term refers to the skin tone color that can be in the color of white, yellow, red or brown.

Basket-Weave Suture: this term refers to the stitches which anchor or hold in place restorative filler that uphold tissues in place.

Beard Area: this term refers to the chin, neck, and lip area where hair grows.

Bilateral: this term refers to two-sided.

Bilateral Silhouette: this term refers to a view which allows comparison of two sides.

Black: this term refers to a color called jet in pigments which indicates an absence of color or hue due to its ability to absorb light.

Blanch: this term refers to a lighten hue of a pale color.

Bleach: this term refers to a chemical which whitens or pales skin discolorations by making color hues lighter or by turning the hues to white.

Blend: this term refers to the mixture or mingling of two or more colors together to make another color.

Blister: this term refers to a pus or water filled bump on top of the skin's surface.

Blotched: this term refers to patches of different color on the skin's surface.

Blonde or Blond: Blonde is the spelling for a female with yellow hair; blond is the spelling used for a male with yellow hair.

Bridge: this term refers to a support that connects two points together like that which you find in between two teeth.

Bronze: this term refers to the copper-like color that is mostly brownish in quality.

Brown: this term refers to a color similar to tanned leather or dirt.

Brilliance: this term refers to a lightness or darkness of an object or color indicating its light quality or brightness.

Brunette: this term refers to a brown hair color of a person.

Bruise: this term refers to an ecchymosis or a discoloration of the skin due to blood leakage after a blow to the body.

Buccal Cavity: this term refers to the space between the lips and gums which forms the entrance to the mouth.

Buccinator Muscle: this term refers to a cheek muscle that retracts the mouth and compresses the cheek in the face.

Bucco-Facial Sulcus: this term refers to a furrow or hollow in the cheek that is vertical in position.

Buck Teeth: this term refers to teeth that are not vertical but jut out at an angle from the mouth from the mandible and/or the maxilla.

Burn: this term refers to that caused by heat, radiation, chemical friction or electricity or extreme cold and is also descriptive of the skin's reaction to the extreme conditions of heat or cold.

Cake: this term refers to the powder pressed into a hard mass used as a cosmetic.

Carbolic Acid: this term refers to phenol which is used as an antiseptic and disinfectant to dry tissues and to bleach discolored tissues of the body.

Carmine: this term refer to a purplish-red color.

Carotene: this term refers to the pigment in skin which is yellowish in color.

Cartilage: this term refers to the elastic substance which attaches muscles to bones and forms parts of the body such as the nose and ears.

Cast: this term refers to a positive production from a negative impression made from a mold.

Caucasian: this term refers to that which relates to white population of the human race.

Caustic: this term refers to a chemical characteristic which causes drying of tissues by searing.

Cement: this term refers to a substance which causes separate surfaces to adhere to each other.

Charred: this term refers to that which has been burned and has a heat-condensed carbon appearance.

Chroma: this term refers to a color purity that is intense in color.

Chromatic Color: this term refers to the visible spectrum colors or the hue of a color.

Cilia: this term refers to the eyelashes of the eye.

Collodion: this term refers to a liquid sealer that is clear and syrupy in texture but dries to a white film consistency.

Colloid: this term refers to the suspension in which pigments are so connected together the particles cannot be separated from each other.

Color: this term refers to a light refraction which separates light's wavelengths with specific attributes of color. Red, blue, and yellow are the primary colors from which all other colors are derived.

Colorant: this term refers to the surface that has been treated cosmetically to produce the color in pigment, dye, paint, or cosmetics.

Colored Light: this term refers to the luminosity which has a visual hue appearance.

Color Filter: this term refers to a substance when light passes through allows certain wavelengths to pass through while absorbing other wavelengths or colors.

Color Wheel: this term refers to a circular item which has an orderly arrangement of hues from primary to secondary to intermediate in color.

Columna Nasi: this term refers to the cartilage in the nose that is between the nostrils of the nose.

Complements: this term refers to any two colors that produce the color gray when mixed together.

Complexion: this term refers to color and texture of the skin in humans.

Component: this term refers to an ingredient of a substance.

Compound Color: this term refers to two or more pigments which makes a different color.

Compound Fracture: this term refers to the bone which is broken and one end protrudes from the skin.

Compress: this term refers to a type of compact dressing of cotton or gauze which is drenched in water or chemical. This dressing is pressed to the skin to preserve, dry, reduce swelling or bleach discolorations of the skin.

Concave: this term refers to the concavity or the hollow in the surface.

Concave Profile: this term refers to the quarter-moon-shaped profile as noted in the forehead and chin which are positioned prominently forward on the body.

Concha: this term refers to the deepest part of the ear known as the concave part of the ear.

Condyle: this term refers to the rounded projection or enlargement of a bone that has segmented surface.

Cones of the Eye: this term refers to the nerves in the eye which sense colors or wavelengths.

Constrict: this term refers to the action that contracts or tightens something.

Contour: this term refers to the surface outline of something.

Contusion: this term refers to a bruise or ecchymosis.

Conversion: this term refers to an illumination color which changes or destroys the color it illuminates or lights up.

Convex: this term refers to the shape that is curved outwardly such as the surface of a ball or other such object.

Convex Profile: this term refers to the facial contour where the forehead and chin are receded more than the superior mucous membrane.

Cool Hue: this term refers to the color leaning towards blue or the portion of light waves in the short length of the spectrum.

Cords of the Neck: this term refers to the part which has vertical prominence.

Corrugator Muscle: this term refers to the muscle that gives movement to the eyebrows.

Cosmetic: this term refers to a substance used for the purpose of covering up imperfections in the skin usually found in the face or neck.

Cosmetic Base: this term refers to a cream or creamy powder foundation which is applied first and used for covering imperfections.

Cosmetician: this term refers to the individual who applies cosmetics to the skin.

Cosmetology: this term refers to the art and study of beautification products for application to improve the appearance and the texture of skin, nails, and hair on the body.

Cranium: this term refers to the head or the part of the skull which encloses the brain in a protective bone.

Cream Cosmetic: this term refers to an emulsion which smoothes on the skin with stroking motions.

Creaming: this term refers to the act of smoothing on a cream or petroleum jelly to massage a surface.

Crest: this describes the position at the apex of a curve.

Cribriform Plate: this term refers to the ethmoid bone that is horizontal and separates the cranial cavity from the nasal cavity.

Crimson: this term refers to a deep color red with a purple tinge.

Crown: this term describes the position at the apex of the head.

Crura: this term refers to the part of the ear that splits in two called the antihelix.

Crus: this term refers to the flattened part of the ear in the concha.

Cuticle Remover: this term refers to a chemical solvent which is used to eliminate dead skin or scabs from the skin.

Decapitate: this term refers to the separation of the head from the body.

Deep Filler: this term refers to a substance which is used to fill a cavity or excisions. This substance also serves as a foundation for surface wax restorations of the body.

Dehydration: this term refers to the removal of water content or a moisture loss of the body.

Dense: this term refers to tightly packed parts.

Density: this term refers to the amount of concentration or the degree of tone or color applied in accordance to the thickness of a cosmetic.

Dental Prognathism: this term refers to a projecting or jutting jaw.

Dental Tie: this term refers to using a thread or wire to hold the jaws together.

Denture: this term refers to artificial of false teeth.

Depress: this term refers to the diminished projection or the force that is used to hold something down into an inferior position.

Depression: this term refers to the forcing down in position or a hollowed out place.

Depressor Angulus Oris: this term also refers to the triangularis muscle which lowers the angle of the mouth.

Depressor Labii Inferioris: this term also refers to the quadratus muscle which pulls the bottom lip lower and in a lateral position.

Depth: this term refers to a degree or level of deepness.

Derma: this term refers to the skin or that which relates to the skin.

Desquamation: this term refers to the point when the body decomposes and the epidermis separates from the dermis and slips from position.

Desiccation: this term refers to the body which is completely devoid of moisture.

Deviation: this term refers to that which is not considered society's norm or that which has been diverted from an accepted way.

Digastricus Muscle: this term refers to the muscle which pulls the hyoid bone forward and backward.

Dilution: this term refers to a watered down or weakened concentration of a solution.

Dimples: this term refers to the concave parts of the cheek which appear and disappear with facial movement.

Disarticulate: this term refers to that which makes the bones become disjoined.

Dissection: this term refers to the action of cutting through or apart.

Distend: this term means to inflate or to swell.

Distortion: this term refers to a warped shape or a shape that is not natural.

Dorsum: this term refers to the ridge of the nose that protrudes or the section that is positioned as the upper surface of the head or body.

Dry Rouge: this term refers to the red powder in a cake form which is used to tinge the skin a pinkish color. This color is usually placed on the cheeks.

Drying Powder: this term refers to the white substance used to remove moisture from a surface.

Dryness: this term refers to the lack of moisture.

Dusky: this term refers to a dark color or a complexion that can be described as swarthy in nature.

Ear: this term refers to the organ which hears sounds.

Ecchymosis: this term is also known as a bruise.

Electric Spatula: this term refers to a heated blade that is used to contour and dry tissues and to reduce swelling of the skin.

Elevation: this term refers to a raised surface.

Elliptical Curve: this term refers to a stretched circle or bow.

Emaciation: absence of fatty tissues due to starvation or illness or wasted appearance of a person.

Embed: this term refers to anchor in a surrounding mass.

Eminence: this term refers to a projection of a bone.

Emollient: this term refers to an agent that softens and smoothes the surface of the skin such as a massaging cream used on the skin.

Emphasis: this term refers to a technique using the same color of light as the object being lighted.

Emulsion: this term refers to the blending of two ingredients which do not blend naturally through the use of a binder or emulsifier.

Epidermis: this term refers to the outer layer of skin on the body.

Ether: this term refers to the flammable, clear chemical used to dissolve wax, remove grease and remove adhesive stains.

Evert: this term refers to that which is in an outward position.

Excision: this term refers to the place from which something has been cut out or removed through the act of cutting out.

Exposed Area: this term refers to portions of the body which remain uncovered such as the hands or the face of the person.

External Auditory Meatus: this term refers to the inferior part of the medial 1/3 of the ear or the ear passage.

External Pressure: this term refers to a pressing down from the outside.

Extraction: this term refers to the removal or the pulling out of something.

Eyebrow Pencil: this term refers to a marker used to enhance the eyebrows with color.

Eyecap: this term refers to a tool used to slip under the eyelid to restore the natural curvature of the closed eye of the facial area.

Eyelid: this term refers to the soft skin flaps which cover and uncover the eyeball of the facial area.

Eye Shadow: this term refers to a color applied to the eyelid of the facial area.

Eye Socket: this term refers to the orbital, bony cavity which holds the eyeball in the facial area.

Face: this term refers to the portion of the head which is defined from the chin to the eyes or hairline.

Facial Markings: this term refers to the indentions, or the small peaks and valleys of the face which appear as wrinkles or dimples or some other marking.

Facial Profile: this term refers to the view of the face from the side.

Facial Proportions: this term refers to the size of facial features to each other and to the head in a mathematical affiliation.

Feather: this term refers to a gradually reduction that tapers away to nothing.

Firmness: this term refers to the tissues which are stable and rigid to the point that wax may be applied.

First Degree Burn: this refers to hyperemia or the condition in which heat or chemicals can cause damage to the skin. The damage suffuses the epidermis and causes redness of the skin.

Florid: this term refers to a complexion which is infused with a red tinge.

Florescent Lamp: this term refers to a source of illumination which uses a low pressure mercury discharge that transfers ultraviolet energy into light.

Fold: this term refers to a prominence which is elongated atop a surface.

Foramen Magnum: this term refers to the half way point between the mastoid processes and the opening in the occipital bone where the spinal cord passes from the brain in the body.

Force: this term refers to a color's ability to draw attention from its intensity or brilliance.

Forehead: this term refers to the part of the head just above the eyes on the body.

Fossa: this term refers to a dip or a concave recess on the body.

Fracture: this term refers to a broken bone in the body.

Frenulum: this term refers to the membrane which connects the upper and lower lips to the gum line of the jaw.

Frontal: this term refers to the anterior or front portion of the body.

Frontal Bone: this term refers to the forehead bone part of the cranium.

Frontal Eminence: this term refers to the prominence or the protrusion in the frontal bone positioned a bit inferior to the center.

Frontal Process of the Maxilla: this term refers to the part of the upper jaw which ascends to the frontal bone as it rises beside the nasal bones of the face.

Furrow: this term refers to the sulcus or wrinkle that appears as a cleft on the face.

Gauze: this term refers to a very loosely woven muslin cloth.

Geometrical: this term refers to the even shapes which are known as the oval, the square, or the circle.

Glabella: this term refers to the portion which is located between the superciliary arched and just above the root of the nose in the frontal bone.

Glycerin: this term refers to a skin softening agent in the form of a liquid that is made from fats or oils and is used in cosmetics.

Gray: this term refers to the black and white pigments that can be combined to make this color in varying degrees of intensity.

Green: this term refers to the mixing of the two primary colors of blue and yellow to produce the secondary color.

Groove: this term refers to an elongated indentation or rut.

Hairline: this term refers to the portion of the scalp where the hair ends.

Hair Patch: this term refers to a replacement article with a number of hairs.

Hard Palate: this term refers to the portion of the roof of the mouth positioned in an anterior spot.

Head Shape: this term refers to the outline of the peripheral part of the head on the body.

Height: this term refers to a vertical measurement.

Helix: this term refers to the outside of the ear.

Hemoglobin: this term refers to the component of red blood cells which carries oxygen through the body.

Highlight: this term refers to the lightest tones in an image or the brightest tone in a room.

Highlighting with Cosmetics: this term refers to a technique in cosmetology which lightens or brightens the complexion of a person.

Horseshoe Curve: this term refers to a U-shape where the ends are narrower than the bottom of the curve.

Hue: this term refers to that which makes colors distinct or intense.

Humor: this term refers to the body fluid which can be of a consistency that is either thin or thick.

Hunting Bow: this term refers to a shape similar to the bent wooden weapon used for hunting animals.

Hypodermic: this term refers to the application or injection beneath the skin.

Illumination: this term refers to light.

Incandescent Light: this term refers to a type of lighting that uses an electric current in a filament to make a light.

Incision: this term refers to the act of precision cutting.

Incisive Fossa: this term refers to the area between the incisor teeth and mental eminence of the facial area.

Incisor Teeth: this term refers to the four teeth that are in the front used for cutting food.

Inclination: this term refers to a tilt or a property of a line that is off vertical and off horizontal.

Indigo: this term refers to a plant dye made synthetically and designated as a deep violet blue which is one of the seven primary colors.

Infantine: this term refers to that which is babyish or childish.

Inferior: this term refers to the lower or underneath portion of something.

Inferior Integumentary Lip: this term refers to the part that is located between the inferior margin of the inferior mucous membrane and the mental eminence.

Interior Nasal Conchae: this term refers to the sidewalls of the nasal cavity which is the lower scroll-shaped bones.

Inferior Palpebral Sulcus: this term refers to the inferior eyelid that is the groove of the inferior border.

Inflammation: this term refers to the swelling and redness found in injured tissues.

Infrared: this term refers to the invisible light on the long wavelength end of the spectrum.

Inhibit: this term refers to the restriction or the slowing down of something.

Inject: this term refers to the forcible introduction of something.

Inner Canthus: this term refers to the medial corner of the eye extension.

Intense: this term refers to the dramatic and vivid color.

Intensify: this term refers to the action to increase a color.

Intensity: this term refers to a color's brilliance moving away from gray or complementary colors.

Interciliary Sulci: this term refers to the furrows between the eyebrows that are vertical.

Intertragic Notch: this term refers to that which is located between the tragus and antitragus of the ear.

Intradermal Suture: this term refers to the hidden suture designed to close incisions without being noticeable to the eye.

Intermediate Hue: this term refers to a color made from mixing primary and secondary colors close together on the color wheel.

Infranasal Prognathism: this term refers to the portion at the base of the nasal cavity.

Inversion: this term refers to the tissues which are turned in an opposite direction or folded in an inward direction.

Inverted Triangle: this term refers to the arrangement where the apex is at the bottom and the base is superior.

Jaw line: this term refers to the inferior part of the chin and jaw of the face.

Juxtaposition: this term refers to the arrangement of two different things side by side or two different colors that modify each other when placed alongside each other.

Labia: this term refers to the lips on the face.

Labial Sulci: this term refers to the vertical grooves of the lips which extend from the mucous membranes into the enveloping layer.

Labiomental Sulcus: this term refers to the junction of the inferior lip and chin which may appear as a furrow on the face.

Laceration: this term refers to an asymmetrical tear in the flesh of the body.

Lanolin: this term refers to oil that comes from sheep.

Lanugo: this term refers to the thin growths of hair which are also known as peach fuzz hair.

Lateral: this term refers to something that is positioned toward the side.

Leak: this term refers to the fluid which escapes or seeps out from an area.

Length: this term refers to a measurement on a vertical plane or surface.

Leptorrhine: this term refers to a high-bridged nose that has an appearance that is long and narrow.

Levator Anguli Oris Muscle: this term refers to the muscle which raises the angle of the mouth.

Levator Labii Superioris Alaeque Nasi Muscle: this term refers to the muscle which dilates the nostrils and raises the superior lip on the face.

Levator Labii Superioris Muscle: this term refers to the muscle which elevates the superior eyelid on the face.

Ligate: this term refers to the action of binding or tying up something.

Ligature: this term refers to the cord or wire used for tying vessels, bones, or tissues of the body.

Light: this term refers to the luminosity or that which the opposite of darkness.

Line of Closure: this term refers to the visible line formed when two structures close or align together.

Linear Sulci: this term refers to the eyelid wrinkles which run horizontally on the palpebrae. These wrinkles may fan from the medial corners and lateral corners of the eyes.

Lip Brush: this term refers to the cosmetic tool used to place color on the lips of the face.

Lip Wax: this term refers to a substance which is used to replace the external mucous membranes of the mouth in the body.

Liquid Cosmetic: this term refers to a base with color used to cover blemishes on exposed flesh or skin.

Liquid Sealer: this term refers to a clear adhesive which dries quickly after application.

Liquid Suspension: this term refers to a liquid with a suspension agent mixed with a powdery substance.

Lobe: this term refers to the lower third of the ear.

Loop Stitch: this term refers to a stitch which anchors or holds restorative materials in place.

Magenta: this term refers to a deep, vibrant purple color that is tinged with reddish tones.

Major Restoration: this term refers to the operations and surgical procedures that take extended amounts of time and requires discussion with relatives beforehand.

Makeup: this term refers to the cosmetics used.

Mandible: this term refers to the bone which is shaped as a horseshoe and forms a person's lower jaw.

Mandibular Fossa: this term refers to the trough in the squamosal bone used for the reception of the mandibular condyle of the teeth.

Mandibular Prognathism: this term refers to the protrusion of the inferior jaw of the face.

Mandibular Sulcus: this term refers to the vertical groove below the jaw line that rises on the cheek.

Mandibular Suture: this term refers to a special stitch which holds the jaw or mouth closed. The special stitch is placed behind the lips, passing around the inferior jaw and through the nasal septum or superior frenulum.

Margin: this term refers to that which is at the edge of the surface.

Mascara: this term refers to a dark, thick fluid used to lengthen and thicken eyelashes around the eyes.

Mask: this term refers to anything that conceals or obscures a view.

Massage Cream: this term refers to a smoothing concoction which is used as a protective coating for the skin.

Masseter Muscle: this term refers to the muscle used for moving the teeth in the act of chewing, grinding, or crushing motions.

Mastoid Process: this term refers to that which is located posterior to the ear and is the rounded projection on the inferior portion of the temporal bones.

Matte: this term refers to the flat finish.

Maxilla: this term refers to the superior jaw or the skeletal base that holds the upper teeth, the roof of the mouth, the nasal cavity sides and the floor of the orbits.

Maxillary Prognathism: this term refers to the part of the upper jaw that protrudes from the face.

Medial: this term refers to that which is positioned in the middle of something.

Medial Lobe: this term refers to that which is located at the midline of the superior mucous membrane as a tiny protrusion.

Melanin: this term refers to the pigment in the hair and epidermis which is light brown to dark brown in color.

Mental Eminence: this term refers to the projection on the anterior mandible which is triangular in shape and form.

Mentalis Muscle: this term refers to the crinkles on the chin's skin and inferior lip that appear as raised, projections.

Mesorrhine: this term refers to a nose which is medium low-bridged and medium broad in shape.

Minor Restoration: this term refers to a procedure which is non-surgical and used to touch up negligible or small areas that show damage.

Mixture: this term refers to a non-chemical reactive blend of two or more ingredients forming one substance.

Modeling: this term refers to that which is formed from a wax or some pliable material into some shape.

Monochromatic: this term refers to that which is only one color.

Mottle: this term refers to a blotchy-type appearance to the skin.

Mouth Former: this term refers to an item used to form the mouth into a natural shape.

Mucous Membranes: this term refers to the lip tissue which is visibly red, having a thin tissue which lines organs and body cavities in contact with air or the exterior environment.

Musculature Suture: this term refers to a closing stitch which holds the mouth shut. This stitch is located behind the lips passing through the muscles next to the inferior jaw and through the nasal septum or the superior frenulum.

Mute: this term refers to a low intensity color which has been toned down by adding on another color.

Mutilated: this term refers to a loss of natural form due to force which causes damage.

Nasal Bones: this term refers to that which is located directly inferior to the glabella and forms a triangular dome over the superior portion of the nasal cavity.

Nasal Cavity: this term refers to a passage way from the nostrils to the back of the throat.

Nasal Spine of the Maxilla: this term refers to the bony projection located midway at the inferior edge of the nasal cavity of the face.

Nasal Sulcus: this term refers to the section between the nasolabial fold and the posterior margin of the wing of the nose.

Nasolabial Sulcus: this term refers to the crinkle in the skin that reaches from the nose to the lateral corner of the mouth of the face.

Nasolabial Fold: this term refers to the protrusion of the cheek which lies adjacent to the mouth next to the sulcus and reaches from the wing of the nose to the corner of the mouth.

Naso-Orbital Fossa: this term refers to the depression superior to the medial portion of the superior palpebrae of the face.

Natural Facial Markings: this term refers to the hereditary features on the face resulting from the birth process.

Natural Shadows: this term refers to the colors in the tissue that are darker than surrounding tissues.

Needle Injector: this term refers to a device which projects metal pins into the bones of the body.

Negative Mold: this term refers to a shaped cavity which gives shape to some type of medium.

Neutral Colors: this term refers to the colors of black, white, or gray.

Nevus: this term refers to the skin discolorations that are found in moles, birthmarks, or blemishes which are present from birth.

Norm: this term refers to that which is common or average.

Notch: this term refers to a deep indentation or gash.

Oblique: this term refers to a tilted or slanted mark which is neither vertical nor perpendicular in nature.

Oblique Palpebral Sulcus: this term refers to the slanted groove which extends from the corner of the eye of the face.

Occipital bone: this term refers to the bone found at the back of the cranium which cradles the brain.

Occipital Protuberance: this term refers to the protrusion at the center of the external surface of the occipital bone.

Occipitofrontalis Muscle: this term refers to the muscle which raises the eyebrows and draws the scalp forward and backward.

Oil-based Cosmetic: this term refers to the makeup that is suspended in an oil base or foundation.

Olive: this term refers to the greenish-tan color having a medium value.

Opaque: this term refers to a light-blocking substance or makeup.

Optic Facial Sulci – this term refers to the wrinkles at the corners of the eyes of the face.

Oral Cavity: this term refers to the mouth found on the face of a person.

Orange: this term refers to a secondary color that is a blend of red and yellow colors.

Orbicularis Oculi Muscle: this term refers to the muscle which squeezes the lacrimal sac and closes the eye lid.

Orbicularis Oris Muscle: this term refers to the muscle which closes the lips.

Orbit: this term refers to the cavity which contains the eye known as the eye socket.

Orbital Pouch: this term refers to the bags under the eyes of the face.

Orifice: this term refers to an opening in the body.

Origin: this term refers to an attachment of a muscle which moves least when the muscle contracts.

Ornamental: this term refers to the purpose of decoration or beauty for esthetic reasons rather than functional purpose.

Oval: this term refers to an elongated circular shape.

Overtone: this term refers to a hue that overlays another color and modifies it as a dominate color.

Palatine Bone: this term refers to the bone which forms part of the nasal cavity that makes up the hard palate of the mouth and part of the orbital cavities.

Palpebra: this term is given for the eyelid of the eye.

Pancake: this term is used for a thick powdery type of makeup.

Parietal Bones: this term is used for the superior portion of the side and back of the cranium as well as the posterior 2/3 of the roof of the cranium.

Parietal Eminence: this term is used for the convex outer surface of the parietal bones.

Paste: this term refers to a mixture that is pliable and useful as a sticky kind of glue.

Patch of Hair: this term refers to a grouping of hairs which are applied to cover missing hair on a person.

Perpendicular Plate of the Ethmoid Bone: this term refers to the superior portion of the bony nasal septum of the face.

Petroleum Jelly: this term refers to a mixture of hydrocarbons which is slick, shiny and semi-solid in texture.

Philtrum: this term refers to the vertical groove located in the middle of the upper lip of the face.

Physiognomy: this term refers to the study of facial features and the surface structure of the face on the body.

Pigment: this term refers to the coloring agent applied through a vehicle of some type.

Pigment Powder: this term refers to coloring agents mixed in the medium of talc.

Pigment Theory: this term refers to the Prang System which has primary colors, secondary colors, and tertiary colors or intermediary colors. Tertiary colors are formed by mixing secondary colors with primary colors. The primary colors are red, blue, and yellow. The secondary colors are red/blue = purple, red/yellow = orange, blue/yellow = green.

Plane: this term refers to a level surface that has no curved shape.

Plaster of Paris: this term refers to a powdery substance called calcium sulfate that when mixed with water, dries hard. This substance is used to encase or set broken bones on a body.

Platyrrhine: this term refers to a short, broad nose that has a low projection.

Platysma Muscle: this term refers to the muscle that depresses the mandible and inferior lip. This muscle crinkles the neck and chest.

Platysmal Sulci: this term refers to the furrow of the neck that dips.

Pledget: this term refers to a ball of cotton or a tuft of fabric.

Plug: this term refers to a gadget that is inserted into a hole which fills the hole with wool, cotton, wood, or some other material.

Point of Entry: this term refers to the place an object enters or penetrates into another object.

Pores: this term refers to the openings of the skin for the sweat glands and oil glands.

Positive Cast: this term refers to the image made from a negative mold or plaster.

Posterior: this term refers to the position at the rear, dorsal, or caudal end.

Postmortem: this term refers to the time after death.

Powder: this term refers to a substance which is ground up into minute particles and is loosely packed.

Powder Atomizer: this refers to a device which can spritz powder on the surface of something.

Powder Brush: this term refers to the tool made of long strands of hair used by a cosmetologist to apply powder to the body.

Powder Puff: this term refers to a soft pad or spherical ball of cotton used to apply powder to the body.

Primary Hue: this term refers to a color that basically red, yellow or blue.

Procerus Muscle: this term refers to a muscle that draws the skin of the forehead inferiorly.

Professional Portrait: this term refers to an image of a person that has special lighting geared to flatter the person.

Profile: this term refers to an outline of the side of a head.

Prognathism: this term refers to a projection of the jaw or jaw line on the face.

Projection: this term refers to a flange, overhang, or protrusion.

Proportion: this term refers to the relationship of features regarding the face or with the length and width of the face on the body.

Protrusion: this term refers to a projection or protuberance.

Puncture: this term refers to a hole made with force that is small in diameter.

Purple: this term refers to a color combination of blues and reds.

Pus: this term refers to a liquid that is formed from inflamed tissue.

Pustule: this term refers to a boil or an abscess.

Pyramid: this term refers to a triangular shape in three dimensions with a broad, square base and an apex at the top.

Quadratus Labii Superior Muscle: this term refers to a muscle which deepens the nasolabial sulcus and raises the wings of the nose on the face.

Radiant Energy: this term refers to electromagnetic waves of various lengths that travel through space.

Radiate: this term refers to a spreading out from a common or central point.

Ramus: this term refers to the part of the mandible which is vertical in position.

Raspberry: this term refers to a dark purplish-red color on the color wheel.

Rat-tail Comb: this term refers to a comb with a long, slender tail which is used to part the hair into neatly combed sections.

Razor Burn: this occurs when the razor removes the epidermis as well as hair on the body.

Reblend: this term refers to the redistribution of a substance into a more uniform density or thickness.

Rectangular: this term refers to an elongated square shape.

Reduce: this term refers to a condensation of size.

Reflection: this term refers to light waves that bounce off an object.

Retrousse: this term refers to a turned up nose.

Rim: this term refers to the top most edge or outermost edge as in the eye socket.

Risorius Muscle: this term refers to the muscle that contracts the angle of the mouth forward.

Rod of the Eye: this term refers to rod-shaped sensors in the retina which respond to light but not colors.

Root of the Nose: this term refers to the top part or the bridge of the nose or the dip inferior to the forehead of the face.

Ruddy: this term refers to the redness in the complexion.

Sallow: this term refers to an unhealthy yellow color to the skin or pallor.

Saturation: this term refers to the deepness of color compared to the degree of difference from gray of the same tones.

Scab: this term refers to a crusty covering of a wound which aids in the healing process.

Scab Oozing: this term refers to a pus, serum or watery substance which seeps out from the wound in or around a formed scab. This usually indicates that an infection is present in the wound.

Scapha: this term refers to that which is located around the outer rims of the ears in a shallow, trench-like depression.

Scarlet: this term refers to a deep, red intense color.

Sealer: this term refers to glue which is moisture resistant after it dries. This keeps any bodily fluids from leaking out of the body.

Sear: this term refers to a searing or burning used to cauterize tissues to provide a dry foundation.

Second Degree Burn: this term refers to the affects of intensive searing or heat to the outer epidermis and the underlying layers of skin. These affects are characterized by pain, redness, swelling and blisters to the damaged areas.

Secondary Hue: this term refers to the combining of two primary colors to form a secondary color.

Septum: this term refers to a thin piece of cartilage, vertically positioned between the two nostrils. This causes one nostril to be larger than the other.

Serrated: this term refers to a jagged cutting edge such as a saw blade.

Sever: this term means to cut off or disconnect from something.

Shade: this term refers to a color description used to indicate different darkness or lightness of one hue from another.

Shadow: this term describes when an object is interfered with regarding a light source and the obstruction of light from another object.

Shampoo: this term refers to the action and the compound used in the cleansing of hair.

Sheen: this term refers to the oils of the face which cause a glossy or shiny look to the skin.

Sideburns: this term refers to the hair that extends from the hairline at the anterior part of the ears down along the jaw line of the face.

Sides of the Nose: this term refers to the lateral walls of the nose on the face.

Simple Fracture: this term refers to a broken bone that does not pierce the skin.

Singe: this term refers to a slightly burned area of skin.

Solvent: this term refers to a liquid in which particles are dissolved.

Spatula: this term refers to a flat-bladed knife used to mix or spread a substance of some type.

Spectrum: this term is used to describe when light is refracted to create visible colors. The complete range from the short wave length blues to the longer wave length reds of color.

Splint: this term refers to a device made from wood or metal which holds the two broken parts of something together.

Spray Cosmetic: this term refers to a substance which is atomized so that it can be rapidly and evenly applied to the skin.

Sponge: this term refers to a porous substance which can usually soak up more than its weight in water or other liquids.

Squama: this term refers to a recession in the temporal cavity of the body.

Square: this term refers to four 90 degree angles connected by sides of equal lengths in a shape.

Stain: this term refers to a discoloration of skin, material or other object by some foreign substance.

Stain Remover: this term refers to an agent which causes the disappearance of discoloration from the flesh.

Sternocleidomastoid: this term refers to the SCM muscle which rotates and pushes down the head of the body.

Stipple Brush: this term refers to a tool with the same sized bristles that is used to simulate pores on wax.

Subcutaneous: this is the term given for the location beneath the skin.

Submental Sulcus: this term is given for the groove located inferior to the junction of the chin and submandibular area of the face.

Subtractive Method: this term is given to the way light is filtered and produces diminishing wave lengths of color transparencies.

Sunken: this term is given for the compressed area or the concave portions of the body.

Superciliary Arches: this term refers to that which is located superior to the median ends of the eyebrows and is positioned at the inferior portion of the forehead of the body.

Supercilium: this term refers to the eyebrows of the face.

Superior: this term refers to the position above or towards the head location.

Superior Integumentary Lip: this term refers to the area positioned between the bottom of the nose and the margin of the upper lip of the face.

Superior Palpebral Sulcus: this term refers to the location of the superior eyelid with a furrow on the upper border of the face.

Supraorbital Area: this term describes that which is located between the supercilium, or eyebrows, and the superior palpebrae of the face.

Supraorbital Margins: this term refers to the superior rims of the eye sockets or orbits of the face.

Surface Filler: this term refers to a substance such as wax used to fill in small depressions in the skin.

Surgical Reduction: this term refers to a procedure which removes swelling by excision after chemicals failed to reduce the swelling's size through the removal of excess moisture.

Suspension: this term refers to the substance which has minute particles floating at the top, but not in a dissolved form.

Sustain: this term refer to that which is held in position by support.

Suture: this term refers to a stitch that holds two ends together.

Swab: this term refers to a tuft of cotton at the end of a short stick used to dab away moisture or applying cosmetics, bleaches or disinfectants substances.

Swarthy: this term refers to a leathery complexion that has been darkened by the sun.

Symmetry: this term refers to evenness to the facial features on each side of the face.

Taper: this term refers to a gradual reduction in size from a central point of something.

Temporal Bones: this term refers to the inferior portion of the sides and base of the cranium, inferior to the parietal bones and anterior to the occipital bone.

Temporal Cavity: this term refers to the depression of the head above the temporal bones.

Temporalis Muscle: this term refers to the strongest chewing muscle that closes and controls the mandible during the grinding of food.

Tenacity: this term refers to the capacity to adhere or to hold onto something.

Termination: this term refers to an end of something.

Tertiary Hue: this term refers to the colors that are combined from secondary colors.

Texturizing Brush: this term refers to a tool that has a large base of fine hairs or bristles used to blend cosmetics.

Third Degree Burns: this term refers to the deepest burn on the under layers of skin which have been seared or charred.

Tints: this term refers to the different quantities of white mixed with one hue or color.

Tinted Powders: this term refers to slightly colored mixtures of pigments and talc or other powdery substances.

Tip: this term refers to the end of the nose or the apex of something.

Tissue Builder: this term refers to a substance used to inflate emaciated tissue or dehydrated tissue to a more normal appearance. This substance is applied by injection with the embalming fluids.

Tones: this term refers to a hue with a dull appearance mixed with a complement or with grays.

Toupee: this term refers to a patch of hair used on the male head that is bald.

Tragus: this term refers to the elevation which protects the ear passage.

Translucent: this term refers to a slightly transparent or frosted unclear treatment.

Transparent: this term refers to a clear, see through texture.

Transverse Frontal Sulci: this term refers to the horizontal wrinkles on the forehead of the body.

Triangle: this term refers to a three-sided form with three angles in the shape.

Triangular Fossa: this term refers to the second deepest depression of the ear.

Turbid: this term refers to a condition which is cloudy or muddy.

Ultraviolet: this term refers to a light of short wavelengths that are not visible to the eye.

Undercoat: this term refers to the foundation that uses pigments or waxes as coverings.

Undercut: this term refers to an incision which is made at an angle.

Unexposed Area: this term refers to the parts and regions which are covered by clothes or other materials.

Value: this term refers to the hue's lightness or darkness of color.

Vehicle: this term refers to the substance in which pigment is contained. Creams, waxes, and fluids are contained in a way that makes applications easier.

Vertical: this term refers to the up and down position which is in opposition to the horizontal position that runs from side to side.

Vitreous: this term refers to the transparent material which is a semi-fluid and is located between the retina and the lens of the eyeball of the face.

Vivid: this term refers to a bright or dramatic color.

Vividity: this term refers to the degree of brilliance that a color has.

Vomer Bone: this term refers to that which is located at the inferior and posterior part of the septum and is on the median plane.

Warm Color Area: this term refers to the colors which lean towards the natural reds found in the skin caused by pink or red pigments.

Warm Hue: this term refers to a color with long wavelengths in the red region of the spectrum of colors.

Wax: this term refers to a material which can be molded and shaped for repairs to the surface of the skin. This is usually comprised of beeswax, spermaceti, paraffin, or starch. The soft skin tone pigments have the ability to reflect light in the same way that living tissue reflects the light.

Weather Line: this term refers to the color change at the margins of wet and dry mucous membranes. One example is found in the line of the lips.

Weight: this term refers to the physical mass which gives the impression of heaviness.

White: this term refers to light which contains all the rays of the spectrum of colors and lack any pigmentation.

White Light: this term refers to the illumination as from the sun which contains all rays of visible spectrum combined into a single ray of brilliance.

Width: this term refers to a measurement of an object from side to side.

Wings of the Nose: this term refers to the lateral lobes of the nose on the face.

Wire Bridging: this term refers to the use of a metal filament to connect two parts that have been broken. The use of a mesh of metal to hold restorative material together is used by embalmers.

Worm Suture: this term refers to a sewing technique which makes sutures invisible from the surface. The edges of the wound are slightly compressed to make the covering of the wound with wax easier. This also makes the appearance more natural to the viewer.

Wound Filler: this term refers to a pliable, doughy-like wax which fills larger cavities for the purpose of repairing wounds or modeling features. This gives a natural appearance to the body.

Zygomatic Arch: this term refers to the portion of the skull which forms the widest part of the face and is located on the temporal bones and zygomatic bones in the facial structure.

Zygomatic Arch Depression: this term refers to the inferior of the zygomatic arch and is a shallow concavity of the face.

Zygomatic Bones: this term refers to the cheekbones that are diamond shaped surfaces located to the inferior sides of the orbits and articulates with the maxilla, frontal, sphenoid and temporal bones of the face.

Zygomaticofrontal Process: this term refers to the lateral end of the frontal bone which is superior to the mandible and anterior to the upper part of the ear on the body.

Zygomaticus Major Muscle: this term refers to the muscle which contracts the superior lip posteriorly, superiorly and anteriorly.

Zygomaticus Minor Muscle: this term refers to the muscle which contracts the superior lip anteriorly and superiorly.

Microbiology

Broad categories

The immune system can be divided into two broad categories. The innate immune system is the first part of the immune system encountered by microorganisms when they invade the body. It can attack any type of pathogen which invades the body. The adaptive, or specific, immune system kicks in after the immune system has been previously attacked and has a type of memory for the next time the same microorganism invades the body. It is considered to be antigen specific. In order to function, both the innate and adaptive immune system are composed of cellular and humoral components.

Immune system cells

The cells which compromise the immune system originate in the bone marrow. These cells are divided into two types: myeloid cells and lymphoid cells. The myeloid cells are subdivided into granulocyte cells (neutrophils, basophils and eosinophils) and monocyte cells (dendritic cells, macrophages and Kupffer cells). The lymphoid cells are divided into three subdivisions: B cells (plasma cells), NK (natural killer) cells, and T cells (cytotoxic cells, helper cells and suppressor cells.) The T cells are released by the bone marrow as precursor T cells. These precursors need to travel to the thymus in order to become T cells. There are two types of T cells: a CD4+ (helper cell) and a CD8+ (pre-cytotoxic.) The helper cells are further differentiated into TH1 cells (which help the CD8+ cells to become cytotoxic T cells) and TH2 cells which help the B cells turn into plasma cells.

Defense mechanisms

There are three main defense mechanisms used by the body to stop pathogens from infecting the host. These are mechanical barriers, humoral barriers and cellular barriers. The mechanical barriers include the skin (shedding of skin cells, mucus production, tears and saliva); chemical reaction of fatty acids, enzymes, surfactants and acidic pH; and biological factors such as normal flora of the digestive system and skin. Cellular components include eosinophils, macrophages, natural killer cells and neutrophils. The humoral response to invading microorganisms activate factors such as interferons, interleukin 1,lactoferrin, lysosomes, and transferrin, and the coagulation and complement systems.

Humoral immunity

The humoral immunity relies upon the triggering of B cells which release large amounts of antibiotics in response to pathogenic invaders such as bacteria or viruses. When a microorganism enters the body, macrophages are activated to engulf and then digest these pathogens. The macrophage then will present antigens from these pathogens on their cell surface. This activates helper T cells to bind to the antigens. These activated T cells will then trigger B cells to multiply and then release antibodies. The antibodies released will then bind to the pathogenic microorganisms to help the body fight off infection.

Cell mediated immunity

Cell mediated immunity begins at birth when stem cells from the bone marrow (lymphocytes) migrate to the thymus gland. While in the thymus, the lymphocytes are processed to be able react to the many different microorganisms which can cause infection in the body. There are three types of T cells: helper T cells, killer T cells, and memory T-cells. The helper T cell will recognize an antigen and present it to lymphocytes in various lymphoid tissues. These lymphocytes will then form into memory cells and killer cells. Helper T cells also attract neutrophils and help macrophages engulf and destroy pathogens. T cell receptor sites on the surface of the T cells will bind to specific antigens. Killer T cells release lymphotoxins which will cause the invading cells to lyse.

Structure of bacteria

Bacteria are considered to be prokaryotic cells which mean they do not have a nucleus. Instead, their genetic material is bound in a nucleoid in the cell's cytoplasm. The cytoplasm will include granules, digestive enzymes, and ribosomes. They have an inner cell membrane. They have a cell wall which protects the bacteria from osmotic pressures. This is where oxidative phosphorylation happens. From the structure of the cell walls the bacteria can be classified into gram positive bacteria and gram negative bacteria. Gram positive bacteria remain stained by crystal violet; gram negative bacteria do not. The peptidoglycan layer in the gram positive bacteria is much thicker than in the gram negative bacteria. Gram negative bacteria also have an extra outer membrane. Between the inner and outer membrane of the gram negative bacteria is the periplasmic space. Other components of the bacteria (varies depending on type) are capsules, pilli, and flagella.

How bacteria reproduce

Bacteria reproduce by one of two methods: asexual reproduction and sexual reproduction. Bacteria which reproduce by asexual reproduction do so by binary fission. The bacteria will make copies of each DNA and then divide itself into two cells. Each cell derived from this method of reproduction is an exact genetic copy of the parent. They can also form "buds" which come off the original cells. Bacteria which reproduce by sexual reproduction are formed via conjugation. During conjugation two bacterial cells will join together and exchange genetic material. Once this genetic material is exchanged the two participants will then undergo binary fission and produce offspring with a new genetic code.

Sterilization versus disinfection

Sterilization is a process used which destroys all living cells, viruses and spores. Objects which are sterilized are done so by the use of heat, chemicals, radiation and/or filters depending upon the physical properties of the item being sterilized. Autoclaves are common devices used to sterilize certain objects through the use of hot steam under high pressure. Disinfection is the process used to remove, inhibit or kill the microorganisms which cause disease. It is done to both objects and the environment. It differs from sterilization in that disinfection will not eliminate all spores or microorganisms but it is usually provides adequate cleanliness levels.

Types of germicides

Microorganisms will be killed by germicides. There are three types of germicides: **disinfectants, antiseptics and chemical sterilants**. Disinfectants will get rid of microorganisms (except for the spores of bacteria) and is used on inanimate objects. Disinfectants will not work well in the presence of organic materials. These will have to be removed in order for the disinfectant to work properly. An antiseptic is used on skin or tissues. It will remove all the pathogenic microorganisms except for bacterial spores. Chemical sterilants will completely remove all microorganisms including spores. Chemical sterilants include liquid chemicals or ethylene oxide gas.

Choosing a germicide

There are a number of considerations when choosing which type of germicide to use. Factors such as object composition will influence choice-steam or high temperature may destroy certain objects so chemical disinfectants may be a wiser choice. Other factors to consider when choosing a germicide include: the shape, surface texture and presence of fissures or cracks; microorganism load; build-up of debris or soil; microorganism resistance; chemical make-up of the germicide; and time exposure and temperature of the germicide. The resistance of microorganisms varies-from order of least resistance to most: viruses, bacteria, fungi, mycobacteria, and bacteria spores.

Bactericidal versus bacteriostatic

Bactericidal is the term used to describe a treatment of a bacterium which ends in killing the organism. Bacteriostatic is the term used to describe a treatment of a bacterium which hinders the organism's ability to grow without necessarily killing it. Treatment methods such as heat (either moist through steam or by the use of dry heat), pasteurization, use of chemicals (gases, solutions, antibiotics), filtration and radiation (ultraviolet light) will be bactericidal. Refrigeration can be bacteriostatic for organisms which cannot reproduce at low temperatures. Freezing or the removal of water or nutrients from the bacterial solution can also be used as bacteriostatic treatments.

Bacterial growth cycle

Bacteria that are growing in optimal conditions will double its population at regular intervals. This is done by exponential growth for a certain part of the bacterial colony life. The growth cycle follows four characteristic phases: lag phase, log (exponential) phase, stationary phase, and death phase. The lag phase begins when the cells are introduced into fresh medium. The population appears to remain static, but the cells are actually increasing in mass, metabolic activity, and are getting ready to divide. During the log phase all the cells are dividing regularly by binary fission. This rate of growth is called generation time (or doubling time). The stationary phase is reached when the population growth is limited due to exhaustion of nutrients, accumulation of waste products, and lack of space. The death phase follows the stationary phase.

Common chemicals used

Common chemicals used to disinfect vary in ability to sterilize and disinfect. Alcohols are medium level disinfectants at 70% concentration. Chlorine mixtures (500-5000mg free chlorine) have high activity of disinfecting. Formaldehyde at 6-8% will sterilize; at 1-8% it will have disinfectant effects. Glutaraldehyde has varying effectiveness (depending on concentration) as a sterilant and disinfectant. Iodophor mixtures at 40-50mg free iodine will have a mid-level disinfectant effect. Peracetic acid at variable concentrations can be a sterilant or a disinfectant. Phenolic mixes at .5 to

3% will have mid to high levels of disinfectant activity. Quaternary ammonium mixtures at .1 to .2% will have a low level of disinfectant activity.

Staphylococcus aureus

Staphylococcus aureus can potentially colonize various areas of the body. The most common sites include the nose, the skin, the gastrointestinal tract, and the perineal area. The nose is a very common area for S. aureus to colonize. People touch their noses quite frequently and pass their S. aureus infection to others by hand contact. Most people will remain asymptomatic carriers of this bacterium; but some people will develop areas of infection (sties, boils, or folliculitis) or wound infection. A huge concern is S. aureus strains which are resistant to antibiotics which are commonly called methicillin-resistant or MRSA strains. These strains are associated with severe necrotizing pneumonia and skin abscesses/infections.

Streptococcus pyogenes

Streptococcus pyogenes is a top pathogen because it causes a number of illnesses including streptococcal pharyngitis, impetigo, acute rheumatic fever, toxic shock syndrome and necrotizing fasciitis. Toxic shock syndrome is any streptococcal infection which causes the body to go into shock and leads to organ failure. This bacterium is a colonizer of the pharynx, especially in children where it will cause pharyngitis on a frequent basis. Most adults that are colonized will be asymptomatic. A protein, streptococcal M protein, helps the bacterium to resist the body's attempt to destroy the organism and it gives the bacterium the ability to multiply in the blood. The M proteins, along with exotoxins, cause massive release of cytokines and lymphokines from monocytes, acting as super antigens during infections.

Anaerobic bacteria

Anaerobic bacteria are bacteria which cannot grow on solid media when there is 18% oxygen or 10% carbon dioxide present. Many important aerobic bacteria can also grow in an anaerobic environment. These bacteria are then called facultative anaerobes. Anaerobic bacteria are extremely common in the human body as components of the normal flora. The gastrointestinal tract, the skin, saliva, the vagina and the periurethral tissues all contain a lot of anaerobic bacteria. They usually do not cause many clinical problems except in these cases: chronic sinus and ear infections, pelvic infections, teeth infections or in people with chronic disease, deep wounds, bowel rupture, necrotic tissues, or in areas of ischemia. Anaerobic infections have characteristics such as the presence of gas or a foul odor.

Transmission of pathogens

Infectious pathogens are transferred from host to others via a variety of means. Contact transmission requires the infected person or object to touch another person or object. Regular hand washing and disinfection of objects will cut down on this type of transmission. Airborne transmission involves the inhalation of fine airborne particles through sneezing or coughing. Infected pathogens remain suspended in air. Masks, covering the mouth and nose when coughing and sneezing, and ultraviolet radiation will decrease this route of transmission. Droplet transmission is the transmission of droplets through coughing, suctioning or sneezing within a three foot radius. Using masks, goggles and shields can reduce the transmission. Vehicle transmission occurs through use of contaminated items (fluids, solutions). Properly discarding contaminated items, proper storage and checking expiration dates will help reduce vehicle transmission. Vector transmission occurs via insects or animals.

Pathogenic organisms

Pathogenic organisms are microorganisms which cause disease in humans and animals. There are many pathogenic organisms: worms, protozoa, fungi, bacteria, viruses and prions. Pathogenic organisms cause the host to become unhealthy through competing with the host for nutrition; destroying cells, tissues and organs; making metabolic products which are toxic to the host; altering body chemistry; inducing the growth of cancerous tissue; or even causing the death of the host. Prions attack the brain tissue. Mad cow disease and Creutzfeldt-Jakob disease are an example of diseases which are caused by prions. Tapeworms and hookworms are examples of worms. Viruses such as influenza, HIV and rabies can cause death in the host. Bacteria such as E. coli or Campylobacter can cause intestinal illness. Fungi such as Aspergillus can cause lung disease. Toxoplasma is a protozoa which can cause illness in new born infants or in people with damaged immune systems.

Transmission of HIV

AIDS is an illness caused by infection with the human immunodeficiency virus (HIV). It is transmitted through the introduction of contaminated body fluid (semen, vaginal secretions, blood and breast milk) into the body through mucous membranes, abrasions, wounds, and blood transfer. The HIV virus attacks several types of white blood cells-in particular helper T lymphocytes (CD4+). The HIV virus DNA is incorporated into the infected lymphocytes. The lymphocytes will begin to reproduce the HIV virus and then eventually become destroyed. The body will then produce enormous quantities of HIV virus so a newly infected person will soon be able to spread the virus to others.

Rickettsia organisms

Rickettsial diseases are caused by bacteria which require a host to live, multiply and survive. These types of infections are spread through insects such as fleas, lice, ticks and mites. When a person becomes infected by a rickettsia organism, the bacteria will infect the endothelial cells of the small blood vessels. These blood vessels will then become inflamed, blocked and will then leak blood into the surrounding tissues. The symptoms of a rickettsial illness are similar: rash, malaise, fever and severe headache. In some cases the disease is much more severe leading to weakness, spleen or liver enlargement, kidney failure, low blood pressure and death. Some diseases caused by rickettsia include typhus, Q fever, and Rocky Mountain spotted fever.

Viruses

Viruses are one of the smallest organisms, smaller than bacteria, which typically have an affinity for a certain cell type. A virus needs to live inside a host's cell in order to reproduce more viruses. It does so by releasing its DNA or RNA when it comes into the cell and forcing the cells to produce copies of the viral DNA or RNA. This will usually kill the host cell, releasing viruses which in turn will go on to infect new cells, repeating the process. Some viruses will not kill the host cell and instead will remain dormant for a long time before becoming active. Other viruses will cause the host cell to replicate repeatedly and become an out-of-control cancerous cell. There are a large number of viruses which cause disease: some common ones include influenza, herpes and Epstein-Barr viruses.

Chlamydia

Chlamydia is primarily a sexually transmitted disease (STD.) Chlamydia trachoma is an obligate, intracellular bacterium which causes trachoma (chronic conjunctivitis), urethritis, cervicitis and genital ulcer disease. It is a fairly common STD and is a primary cause of infertility in females. In addition, it cause pelvic inflammatory disease in women, epididymitis in men and in women can cause infection around the liver. However, most people will remain asymptomatic and will not be aware that they have the disease. It is fairly common for both men and women to be co-infected with gonorrhea when they have Chlamydia. Newborn infants can become infected as they pass through the infected birth canal of their mothers. This infection can cause conjunctivitis in the infant and also pneumonia.

Protozoa

A protozoon is a free-living, unicellular eukaryotic organism which usually does not cause human illness. However, some will cause health problems if they enter a human host or if protozoa affect the environment in some manner (i.e. red tides). There are some protozoa which cause human disease. Naegleria fowleris will cause acute primary amebic meningoencephalitis. Acanthamoeba spp. will cause skin, lung and eye disease and can cause chronic granulomatous amebic encephalitis. Balamuthia mandrillaris can cause granulomatous skin and lung disease. Red tides will produce toxins which accumulate in the fatty tissues and organs of fish and shellfish and when consumed by humans will cause illness.

Important terms

Bacillus anthracis: this term refers to the bacteria pathogen that causes anthrax. Anthrax causes spores to enter a wound through inhalation. Skin lesions, flu-like symptoms, cyanosis, shock, disorientation, coma, and respiratory failure can occur.

Bordetella pertussis: this term refers to the bacteria pathogen that causes whooping cough. Droplets are inhaled that contain the bacteria resulting in violent coughing spells interspersed with a whooping sound when sucking in air.

Borrelia burgdorferi: this term refers to the bacteria pathogen that causes Lyme disease through a tick bite resulting in CNS infection or heart infection.

C. perfringens: this disease is caused by intoxicated food. Signs include gas gangrene and post mortem tissue gas. Symptoms from the disease result in abdominal pain, diarrhea, and necrosis when the bacterium ferments carbohydrates in the gut and promotes decomposition.

C. tetani: this term refers to the bacteria pathogen that causes lock jaw or tetanus. Contaminated soil enters a wound resulting in muscle contraction and respiratory system failure.

Campylobacter jejuni: this term refers to the bacteria pathogen that causes intestinal ulcers when the bacterium is ingested resulting in bloody diarrhea and flu-like symptoms in a person.

Childbirth Fever: this disease is caused by contaminated instruments or hands resulting in infection of the uterus. It can spread to the peritoneum and cause peritonitis leading to death.

Clostridium botulinum: this term refers to the bacteria pathogen that causes botulism when toxins are ingested resulting in paralysis, respiratory system failure, heart failure, double vision, stomach sickness, and swallowing difficulties.

Contamination: results when an infectious organism becomes present on a body surface, inanimate objects such as bedding or instruments, or in food, water or milk.

Corynebacterium diptheriae: this term refers to diphtheria which results from inhaling droplets or hand to mouth ingestion causing throat inflammation, fever, fatigue, neck swelling, forming of pseudo-membrane in pharynx, demyelization of the PNS, and paralysis. Traveler's Diarrhea: this term refers to bacteria ingested from contaminated water or food which causes flu-like symptoms, diarrhea, and cramps.

Endotoxin: is a part of the outer membrane of certain gram negative bacteria. They can cause shock and fever, but are not as potent as exotoxins.

Escherichia coli: this bacterium is known as Enteroinvasive E. coli or enterohemorrhagic E. coli and occurs from fecal-oral ingestion resulting in cramps, general out-of-sorts feeling, pus-filled diarrhea with mucous and blood, kidney failure, fever, and anemia.

Exotoxin: this is a substance produced by bacteria (either gram negative or gram positive) which causes injury to the host cells. It is formed within the cell which releases it into the environment. It only takes a small amount of exotoxin to cause deleterious effects.

Francisella tularensis: this term refers to rabbit fever or tularemia which occurs through inhaling, ingestion, or bites where bacteria enters a wound from a deer fly, tick or rabbit lice bite resulting in a small ulcer locally with inflammation, lymph node enlargements, pneumonia and abscesses over the body.

Haemophilus influenzae: this term refers to influenzal meningitis caused by respiratory droplets resulting in stiff neck, fever, headache, arthritis and pneumonia in a person.

Helicobacter pylori: this term is known as peptic and gastric ulcers caused by ingestion of bacteria resulting in nausea, vomiting, and a burning feeling in the abdomen.

Hypersensitivity: this is an abnormal sensitivity in a body in which a foreign substance stimulates the body to cause an extreme response to the substance.

Infection: An infection occurs when a pathogenic organism gains entry to a host, draws nourishment from the host, multiplies and causes deleterious effects to the host.

Infestation: this occurs when a pathogenic agent (lice, mites, insects) becomes established on (as opposed to in) a body.

Klebsiella pneumoniae: this is a nosocomial respiratory infection caused by bacteria inhaled as droplets resulting in urinary tract, respiratory system and wound infections.

Legionella pneumophila: this is also known as Legionnaires' disease caused by Legionella an airborne bacteria resulting in symptoms of pneumonia, fever, and cough.

Leptospira interrogans: the bacteria Leptospirosis enters through the skin which contacts contaminated water, soil or animal waste resulting in muscles aches, chills, fever, headache, CNS infection, renal and hepatic infection.

Listeria monocytogenes: this term refers to the bacteria Listeriosis caused by bacterial ingestion which results in diarrhea, nausea, stiff neck, fever, body aches, confusion, and convulsions.

M. tuberculosis: this is a form of tuberculosis caused by bacteria droplets resulting in bloody sputum, cough, chest pain, weight loss, anorexia, chills, fever, night sweats, and a general weakness of the body.

Meningococcal Meningitis: this bacterium is contracted through respiratory droplets or direct contact resulting in headache, fever, rash, spontaneous blood clotting, stiff neck, and Waterhouse-Friderichsen Syndrome.

Mycobacterium avium: this is also known as MAC or mycobacterium avium complex which is idiomatic. It is assumed that this bacterium is acquired environmentally and results in weight loss, fever, chills, night sweats, swollen glands, abdominal pain, diarrhea, and weakness. It is usually found in people with fewer than 50 T4 cells.

N. meningitides: this term refers to the Ophthalmia neonatorum bacterium which is contracted in the birth canal resulting in infant blindness.

Neisseria gonorrhoeae: this is also known as Gonorrhea and is contracted through direct sexual contact. The result is a pus-like discharge from the genital tract, sterility, rectal infections, and pain when urinating.

Otitis Media: this infection is caused by bacterial contaminated water, eardrum puncture, or skull fracture resulting in earache caused by pus behind the ear drum.

Pneumococcal Pneumonia: this disease is caused by inhaling droplets resulting in fluids in the lungs, fever, chills, dyspnea, chest pain and bloody sputum.

Proteus Species: this bacterium is found in infected burns caused by a contamination through the wound.

Proteus vulgaris: this bacterium is found in general decomposition caused by bacterial translocation resulting in putrefactive bacteria formed amines.

Rheumatic fever: this term refers to the bacterium found in droplets from strep throat. Rheumatic fever bacteria may lay dormant for years before injuring the mitral valve. In most cases, it can lead to endocarditis and infection of multiple layers of the heart resulting in cardiac failure.

S. pyogenes: this bacterium is found in impetigo caused by an insect bite or through a wound or abrasion resulting in blisters that turn into leaking lesions and crusty sores when the lesions dry up.

S. typhi: the bacteria causing typhoid fever is ingested by the fecal-oral route resulting in fever, headache, whitish fur-like growth on the tongue, rose colored spots on the abdomen, and nose bleeding.

Salmonella enteritidis: Salmonella food poisoning is caused by ingestion of contaminated food resulting in fever, chills, abdominal pain, and diarrhea.

Scarlett Fever: this term refers to the bacterium found in droplets that cause sore throat, red rash, fever, spotted tongue, shedding of the skin lesions, and tongue membrane loss.

Septic sore throat: this disease caused by strep throat caused by exposure to droplets and close contact to the bacteria. It results in soreness in throat, malaise, fever, headache, nausea, vomiting, and abdominal pain.

Shigella: this bacteria (also known as gay bowel syndrome or shigellosis) causes dysentery after exposure via the fecal-oral route by anal-oral contact, sex, flies, fingers, and contaminated food or water. It results in diarrhea with blood and mucous, cramps and fever of the body.

S. pneumoniae: this bacterium is found in pneumococcal meningitis caused by droplets resulting in headache, stiff neck, and fever.

St. Vitus' dance: this term is also known as Sydenham's chorea which is characterized by uncontrollable jerky movements of face, arms or legs.

Staphylococcus aureus: this bacterium is found in skin infections and wound infections caused by direct contact resulting in pimples, furuncles, carbuncles, and septicemia.

Streptococcus agalactiae: this bacterium is found in newborn meningitis caused by the ingestion of raw milk resulting in lethargy, jaundice, breathing distress, anorexia, pneumonia, and shock.

Toxic Shock Syndrome: this is caused by the use of tampons or by surgery resulting in a fever, rash, dehydration, diarrhea, vomiting, hypotension, or shock.

Treponema pallidum: this bacterium is found in syphilis and is caused by direct sexual contact resulting in chancre, rash, blindness, and CNS infection.

Vibrio cholerae: this bacterium is found in Asiatic cholera and is caused by contaminated seafood resulting in a rice-water stool, increase in blood viscosity, and shock to the body.

Virulence: this is a measurement of a disease producing agent's ability to cause a severe illness. It is usually expresses as a ratio of the number of cases to the total number of infections.

Yersinia pestis: this bacterium is found in Bubonic plague caused by flea bites, infected animals, and airborne pathogens, resulting in dark discoloration of the body from hemorrhages and buboes on the lymph nodes.

Pathology

Types of pathology

Pathology is the study of suffering which integrates a clinical viewpoint of its principles. Pathologists study both the cause and symptoms of diseases within the body. General pathology places the center of attention upon cellular and tissue deterioration. Morbid anatomy is the study that is concerned with the body's structure changes. Gross pathology studies diseases and the physical changes seen with the eye. Microscopic pathology or histopathology studies the cell, the tissues, and the organs for changes at the microscopic level. These changes are caused by disease. Surgical pathology is the study of tissue that has been removed by surgery. Clinical pathology is the study of how disease affects bodily fluids. Physiological pathology determines how disease affects bodily functions. Forensic pathology or medicolegal is the study of disease which causes death. Forensic pathology is also concerned with the modes of death.

Purposes of autopsy procedure

Autopsies are performed for several purposes. The first purpose is to identify the condition of the body at the time of death. The second purpose is to establish the how, then when, and the way that death occurred. The third purpose is in the identification of diseases, anomalies, and any other internal or external factors that should be noted. The fourth purpose is to record the internal and external injuries of the deceased. The fifth purpose is the extraction of samples for reasons of microbiological or histological assessments. The sixth purpose is for the collection of evidence in the organs and tissues of the deceased. The last purpose is in the analyses of the findings for interpretation by an expert. A funeral director understands the functions and conditions left by an autopsy as they help the survivors cope with loss. This information is useful in the preparation of the body.

Autopsy components

The components of an external autopsy include examination of the body to detect certain physical conditions. The body is examined to determine: sex, race, hair/eye color, height, weight, external markings such as tattoos, contusions, deformities, scars, amputations and any other physically observable attributes that may be needed to identify the person. In addition, samples of vomit, blood, body fluids, evidence of sexual activity, and/or other foreign matter are collected. Post mortem internal examinations begin with a Y shaped incision at each shoulder and down the torso. The internal organs are uncovered and removed, or partially removed, for examination purposes. The viscera may be put in a viscera bag and returned to the body. The brain is almost always removed by posterior incision in the scalp with an autopsy saw. Empty body cavities may be filled with absorbent materials.

Common diseases

Disease is defined as an illness that can be associated with pain, distress, and suffering to an individual. Some diseases have definite external physical symptoms. Organic disease manifests definite bodily changes as in chicken pox. Hereditary disease is on a genetic level and is transferred from parent to child. Congenital disease is present at the birth of an infant. An acquired disease is contracted after birth. However, some diseases are only noticeable on molecular levels. Some examples of these types of disease are found in person's suffering from high blood pressure or schizophrenia. Communicable diseases are ones that are spread directly or indirectly among the human population. Endemic is an ever-present disease in a community of people. A pandemic is a wide-spread or worldwide disease which is spread through some type of contagion as in the HIV virus. Idiopathic diseases have unknown causes.

Injury and cellular changes

Normally cells will work to maintain a state of homeostasis. However, when a cell is unable to maintain a proper balance in osmotic pressure, then swelling of the cell can occur. Certain adverse conditions can have an effect on the human cells. These changing conditions within the environment can be created as a result of a lack of oxygen, drug or alcohol abuse, infections, immunological reactions, obesity or starvation, trauma, extreme temperatures, radiation, or electric shock. The cells react to the change in environment by striving to achieve the homeostasis. Swelling is the result. The embalmer can sometimes reduce the swelling by introducing hypertonic solution to the body. Hypertonic solutions have a higher pressure than the cell and can cause the cell to shrink in a process called crenation. The use of a hypotonic solution will cause the cells to swell as it has a lower pressure.

Embalming process challenges

Embalmers must be familiar with the universal body changes from cancer such as edema, blood clotting, vascular damage, dehydration and emaciation. Changes hinder the embalming fluid flow into the veins and capillaries. This results in quick bacterial growth, decomposition, or unsightly tissue swelling. In addition, diminished circulation from clots, tumors, or emboli can present a blockage in the vein which inhibits the proper flow of the embalming fluid. Dehydration before death may leave places in the body that are emaciated. An edema can restrict the body's immune system from protecting itself against agents causing infection and abscess. After death a very rapid decomposition in the body can occur. Staining or discoloration from bruises and hematomas can be difficult to disguise. Hemorrhages can cause embalming fluid to enter extravascular tissues creating local swelling, especially in the soft tissue around the eyes.

Tuberculosis risk

Mycobacterium tuberculosis is a term which refers to an aerobic microbe or MTB. This is a very slow growing bacterium which generally affects the lungs of an infected person. The disease is called Tuberculosis (TB). TB can also attack the central nervous system, lymphatic system, circulatory system, genitourinary system, bones and joints. This disease is prominent in third world countries and a large number of the population die from this disease. However, a rise in the numbers infected in developed countries can be traced to loosely controlled populations of infected immigrants coming into the developed countries. Transmission of this disease comes from the MTB in the body fluids expelled when an infected person sneezes, coughs, spits, speaks or blows the nose. Each droplet can contain 2-3 bacilli which is contagious. Studies show embalmers were twice as likely to be reactive to tuberculin as non-embalmers.

Prefixes

a--without
acro--extremity
adeno--gland
an—without
ante—before
anti—against
arthro—joint
auto—self
bio—life
chol—bile
cyst—bladder
dia—through
dys—difficult
en—in
endo—within
entero—intestine
epi—upon
ex—out of
hem, hemo—blood

hetero—dissimilar
homeo—similar
hydro—water
hyper—above or excess
hypo—deficiency or beneath
hyster—uterus
infra—below
inter—between
intra—within
leuko—white
macro—large
mal—bad
mast—breast
mega—great
melan—thick
men—month
micro—small
myo—muscle

myx—mucus
necro—death
neo—new
nephr—kidney
oligo—few
osteo—bone
peri—around
phago—to eat
phleb—vein
polio—grey
poly—many, excess
post—after
pro—before
pseudo—false
pyo—pus
syn—together with
xanthro—yellow

Suffixes

algia—pain
angio—vessel
ase—enzyme
cele—protrusion
centesis—perforating
chole—bile
ectasis—dilate
ectomy—removal of
emesis—vomit
emia—blood
esthesia—sensation
genesis—generation of
iasis—a process

itis—inflammation of
lith—stone
lysis—to dissolve
malacia—softening
megaly—large
odynia—pain
oid—like
oma—tumor
osis—full of
ostomy—mouth
otomy—cut
pathy—disease
penia—poverty, decrease

phila—affinity for
plasia—to form
plegia—paralysis
pnea—breath
ptosis—falling
rhagia—bursting forth
rhea—flow
sclerosis—hardening
statis—standing still
trophy—nourish
uria—relating to urine

Universal Precautions

The Universal Precautions were recommended by the CDC in 1990. However, in 1991 they were required by OSHA. All human remains must be treated as though the remains were infected with contagions. Funeral service workers must wear face shield, gloves, full-length gown, head covering, and shoe coverings. Linens must be laundered between usages and a use of topical disinfectants must be used on the decedent, clothing and removal cot. Prevent aerosolization of microbes by carefully handling clothing and personal effects. Drainage tubes and a closed drainage system prevents body fluid spatter. Body fluid spills should be cleaned up immediately. Medical hazardous waste disposal system for sharp objects and biohazardous waste should be strictly adhered. Disinfect all work surfaces, equipment and the floors of the area. Finally, the embalmer should shower after embalming. Washing of the hands should be done before the embalmer exits the embalming room

Pathogen transmission methods

A reservoir is that which houses the pathogen before transmittal to a host. There are at least two transmission methods of disease causing pathogens used. Direct transmission has three means: physical contact, droplet infection, and congenital transmissions. Person to person contact is the general means of transmission through either a casual or an intimate touch. The virulence of the microbe determines how close the contact must be before transmission can occur. Fecal-oral is transmitted through the shaking of hands and sexual contact. The best defense is good hand washing. Sexual transmissions are accomplished when the pathogens survive in warm, moist environments. Mothers can spread disease to their fetuses. Any blood-to- blood contact can result in transmission of disease which makes embalmers at high risk for infection. Indirect transmission includes food, drink, fomites, water, soil, and both biological vectors and mechanical vectors. Animals and insects can also be carriers.

Postmortem conditions

Tumors
Oncologists study tumors or neoplasms in a science called oncology. Tumors can be cancerous or benign. Cancer is the leading cause of death. These seven common post mortem conditions exist in cancer related deaths: a) Emaciation; b) Dehydration; c) Cachexia; d) Discoloration; e) Hemorrhage; f) Tissue deformation; and g) Extravascular obstructions. Embalmers can expect to find excess fluid around the tumor, loss of hair or alopecia, jaundice, blood clotting disorders, and prosthetic devices. Cachexia occurs when the body wastes away. Atrophy of tissues or emaciation can be due to starvation. Tissue builder injections can be used around the facial hallows such as the eye orbits and around the temples. Both benign and malignant tumors can inhibit the embalming process because growths block blood vessels. Malignant tumors can cause extreme tissue deformation and damage because they infiltrate as they grow and these deformations may entail extensive restorative art techniques.

Congestive heart failure
Congestive heart failure can impact multiple body systems because the heart is not able to pump as much blood as needed. This can engage the left side, the right side or the whole heart. After diastole, some blood remains in the ventricles. Not enough blood enters the arteries. Fluids build up in the tissues which become edematous and weaken the heart. Right-sided heart failure is a disorder of the left ventricle. Right sided heart failure produces severe edema in the hands, feet and abdomen or anasarca. Chronic right-sided heart failure leads to enlarged abdominal organs like the liver. Left-sided heart failure is caused by high blood pressure, mitral or aortic valve diseases, coronary artery disease and myocardium diseases. Pulmonary edema ensues from LSHF, shortness of breath or dyspnea, a reduction of blood in the kidneys, and congested blood clots. These conditions can lead to stroke or coronary artery blockages.

Uremia
Urotropin is formed when nitrogenous waste products are present in the blood. When this comes in contact with formaldehyde, then copious amounts of formaldehyde are needed. The large amounts of formaldehyde are needed to overcome the neutralizing effect of the nitrogen in the blood. Jaundice embalming fluids should be used because of the buffers they contain. The buffers in the jaundice embalming fluids counteract the pH-altering nitrogenous waste products. The

benefits are also found in the cosmetic results of this product. Formaldehyde cross-links proteins and contact with nitrogenous waste to slow down or stop the process. This is due to the altered protein structures in nitrogenous waste-filled tissues.

Reproductive disorders

Blood coagulation will inhibit the absorption of embalming fluids. Ascites is the fluid found in the abdomen that can cause purge from the mouth, nose and ears. Microbes that cause infections require proper disinfectant usage to eliminate the possibility of purge. Infections can include sexually transmitted diseases which can be commuted to the embalmer if the proper procedures are not followed. Lesions must be topically disinfected. Hyperdermically applied preservatives are strongly recommended. Lesions also may cause discoloration and deformations which require repair. In males, hydrocele or the swelling of the scrotum and testicles due to accumulation of fluid can be present. This condition requires deep aspiration of the scrotum and a heavy injection of cavity embalming fluids. Puncturing the scrotum should be avoided because that may cause leakage. The male genitals should be covered with embalming powder after the anus is packed and the whole should be covered with absorbent cotton.

Endocrine system disorders

Excessive fluids will dilute the preservation of the embalming fluids. Any endocrine system disorder in a decedent may require several injection points with several different levels of concentration. One condition that causes a rash like stain is found in the Waterhouse-Friderichsen Syndrome. Hemorrhaging can inhibit the work of the embalmer. Necrosis and massive congestion of the blood may also be a factor which inhibits the dispersion of the embalming fluids. The deceased may have been a sufferer of Addison's disease. This may prevent the embalmer from using high concentration of embalming fluids. To do so would cause darker discoloration of visible areas on the decedent, especially around the face. The embalmer more than likely will not be able to use embalming solutions to fix the deformities caused by the endocrine disorders. However, the embalmer can use proper positioning to prepare the body.

Important terms

Abatement: Reduction in symptoms or reduced pain in a person.

Abdominal distention: Excessive fluid, microbes, and/or malignant tumor in the abdomen which causes the stomach to bulge.

Abscess: Area walled off by a membrane. The area is full of pus which is a protein enriched fluid packed with white blood cells (neutrophils) and cell waste. The membrane shields the surrounding tissue from any more injury or damage.

Acapnia: Reduction of carbon dioxide presence in the blood in the body.

Acidosis: The marked presence of acid in the blood.

Active hyperemia: this term is used for the pathological condition that results from an inflammatory disease. Evidence of inflammation can be seen in the redness, heat, or swelling found in the area.

Addison's disease: A disease of the adrenal glands which gives skin a bronze discoloration most visible in scars, lips, mucous membranes and pressure points (elbows, knees etc). Concentrated formaldehyde is not recommended for this condition because it may cause darker discolorations.

Adenoma: The glandular epithelium or the secretion of cells which produce tumors in the body.

Alkalosis: The marked presence of alkali in the blood stream.

Alzheimer's disease: A progressive and not reversible decline in mental capacity. There is no cure and it is idiopathic in nature. Dr. Alois Alzheimer noticed starch-like material called amyloid plaques and neurofibrillary tangles in a woman's brain. She died of a mental disorder. This condition also causes nerve damage in the area of the brain that controls memory and brain functionality and a reduction in brain chemicals or neurotransmitters required for cell communication. Autopsy is the only way to diagnose this disease. Treatment is with drugs which help reduce the symptoms, but do not provide a cure.

Amelia: A baby that is born without limbs or extremities.

Anasarca: A severe edema.

Anemia: Blood that lacks the ability to transport oxygen or the blood's capability is decreased because of a decreased number of red blood cells.

Aneurysm: Enlargement of an artery due to weakness or injury of the vessel.

Angioma: A hemangioma or neoplasm due to blood vessel dilations.

Aplasia: When a baby is born without one or more organs or when the blood becomes non-regenerative.

Aplastic Anemia: Improper growth or inhibited function of bone marrow. Chemical agents, X-rays and radiation cause bone marrow damage to the extent that it is unable to produce enough red blood cells. Blood cells contain hemoglobin which is the molecule that carries oxygen to the tissues of the body.

Apoplexy: Also known as a stroke. This occurs when a blood vessel that brings blood to the brain bursts. The result is a lack of blood going to the brain tissue and when this happens, the tissue dies.

Appendicitis: Inflammation of the vermiform appendix within the body. This can cause the appendix to burst and be fatal if peritonitis develops. It is idiopathic in nature.

Arrhythmia: Lack of the normal, rhythmic beating of the heart. When fibrillation and arrhythmia occur simultaneously, sudden death occurs.

Arteriosclerosis: Hardening of the arteries and loss of elasticity. It takes two forms: sclerosis of arterioles and the calcification of the medial layer of the arteries.

Arteritis: Inflammation of the arteries and is mostly idiopathic. Two types are Temporal and Takayasu's which occur mostly in Asian women.

Arthritis: A joint disease. It accompanies edema which is extravascular and cannot generally be removed by the arterial embalming process.

Ascites: Digestive disorder that manifests as the accumulation of serous fluid in the abdomen cavity.

Ascites: Excess fluid in the abdomen of the body.

Asphyxia: When insufficient oxygen causes loss of consciousness in a person.

Asthma: This disorder occurs when the irritated mucous lining of the bronchi causes the bronchi to swell shut reducing airflow. Allergens, food, and infections can cause an attack.

Atelectasis: The "incomplete expansion" of a lung, or what is commonly known as a collapsed lung. The lung can be either obstructed or non-obstructed.

Atherosclerosis: The fatty substance deposits which accumulate in the inner lining of the artery called plaque fragmentation.

Atrial Septal Defect: When the foramen ovale fails to close in newborn infants. The right ventricle and the lungs are circumvented by too much blood because of the hole in the interatrial septum. This causes a lack of oxygenated blood in the system and is the cause of "blue baby". Deficiency of oxygen in the tissues gives the baby a blue hue.

Avulsion: A wound caused by the sudden tearing or ripping away of skin.

Bacteremia: Bacterial infection that is located in the blood.

Benign: Type of tumor which is not cancerous or progressive. It does not spread to surrounding tissue in usual cases. However, these tumors do grow and expand and can cause serious disease and death.

Bilirubin: Red pigment in bile which is produced by a chemical breakdown of hemoglobin.

Biliverdin: Green pigment in bile produced by a chemical breakdown of hemoglobin.

Biological Transmission: Occurs when the pathogen requires the mosquito to go though one or more stages to maturity to be spread.

Breast cancer: A lump found in the female breast. A biopsy is required to determine if the breast has a malignant tumor. This is done with fine-needle suction or use of a larger needle that can remove larger tissue or cell samples.

Bronchitis: This disorder affects the air passages to the lungs called the bronchi. The two types are acute and chronic. Chronic is mostly due to inflammation rather than infection or microbes. Acute begins with infection and can be caused by both bacteria and viruses.

Bursitis: Inflammation of the bursae which cushion the pressure points in joints.

Carbuncle: A deep-seated abscess which is usually caused by infection of several contiguous hair follicles.

Carcinoma: Used to generally describe cancer or a malignant neoplasm in a person.

Cardiomyopathy: Restrictive - lower chambers of the heart are rigid and do not expand as ventricles fill with blood; causes are unknown, but may include fat/protein build-up, excess iron, radiation exposure, connective tissue diseases, heart attack, scar tissue. Dilated - left ventricle is enlarged and stiff, causes decreased ejection of blood from the heart; inherited or derived from coronary artery disease, alcoholism, thyroid disease, diabetes, viral infection, valve abnormalities, drugs that are toxic to the heart. Hypertrophic - heart muscle thickens usually in the left ventricle below the aortic valve; walls of the heart harden and there is abnormal valve function; can be hereditary, may also be due to high blood pressure or the aging process.

Cellular infiltration: Reaction to injury on a cellular level which may lead to the presence of pigmentation, calcification, or gout in a person.

Cerebral Edema: Nervous system trauma that leads to death. The blood or other brain barrier prevents embalming fluid from entering the brain tissue. When the lymphatic drainage of edematous fluid is inhibited by hemorrhage or other blockage, the addition of embalming fluids may distend or deform the decedent's head. Proper drainage before embalming will prevent purge and the malformation of the head.

Cerebral Stroke: A cerebral blood vessel that bursts and causes internal bleeding. The third leading cause of death in America is the result of a stroke. Adults who smoke or have factors including hypertension, diabetes mellitus, or high cholesterol are at greater risk. The term "brain attack" is becoming more prevalent among lay persons.

Chancre: The first indication of syphilis in the form of a lesion or sore on the skin.

Chemotaxis: White blood cells that swarm into the wounded site area like cops to surround the micro-foreigners within the cell.

Cholangitis: Inflammation of the bile duct in the body. Acute infection of the bile duct causes blockage of the duct and the mortality rate is high.

Cholecystitis: Inflammation of the gall bladder within the body.

Cholelithiasis: Gallstone formation and inflammation of the gallbladder. This is caused by crystallized bile in the bile duct or in the gallbladder.

Cholelithiasis: this term refers to the presence of gall stones which can cause pain.

Circulatory Shock: An insufficient blood flow which results in inadequate O2 distribution to cells of the body. Without sufficient blood pressure, the body's tissues starve for oxygen and death occurs. All types of circulatory shock exhibit one or more stages: 1. nonprogressive or compensated stage; 2. progressive stage; and 3. irreversible stage.

Cirrhosis: A degenerative liver disorder which has been caused by alcoholism, poison, or hepatitis.

Coagulase: The enzyme which helps the blood to clot. The enzymes help bacteria to use the blood as a nutritional source.

Colitis: Inflammation of the colon within the intestines.

Compensated Stage: A mild drop in pressure in order for the body to restrict its vessels and increase its heart rate. This type of compensating will result in a reduced blood flow in the body.

Concussion: Injury to the head caused by blunt force trauma or other types of trauma. It may be caused by fractures in the skull bone, but that is not necessarily the case. It results in temporary consciousness loss, vomiting, seizures, paralysis and possible memory loss.

Contusion: Caused by traumatic injury to the head and is a more severe condition than a concussion because it is accompanied by hemorrhaging. This is trauma of sufficient force to bruise the brain. This can happen without rupturing the meninges and can occur at any point of the head. Sometimes the point of trauma is not where the contusion occurs, such as when the blow is to the back of the head from falling backwards, the contusion can be on the frontal lobe because the brain is slammed against the front part of the skull.

Copious Blood Disorders: The three disease groups: red blood cells, white blood cells or bleeding disorders.

Coronary Artery Disease: An ischemic heart disease which commonly causes death. It is due to atherosclerosis or a hardening of arteries. Its severity is attributed to three changes: acute plaque changes, blood clots, and spasms of the coronary artery.

Crohn's Disease: Inflammation of the intestines. It is idiopathic. Complications include arthritis, skin problems, kidney stones, gallstones, disease of the liver and biliary system.

Cyanosis: Blue discoloration of the skin which denotes the presence of deoxyhemoglobin. This condition is removed by embalming fluids, but the fluids must be adequate and properly disbursed. The complete removal of cyanosis may require gentle massage and non-astringent arterial embalming fluids depending upon postmortem interval.

Cyst: A fluid or air-filled sac which is either on the body or in the body. Ovarian cyst: this term refers to a fluid-filled sac on the ovary. This occurs in 50% of women who have intermittent menstrual cycles and in 30% of women with regular cycles. Generally, they are not painful, and usually benign. Pressure is exerted on surrounding organs and there can be some twisting of the ovary and may need surgical removal. They can be present at birth or develop during child-bearing years or even later. They cause an acutely sharp pain when they rupture or burst.

Cystitis: A bladder infection. Interstitial cystitis is idiopathic and there is currently no cure for it.

Dehydration: Loss of fluid in the body resulting in a lack of fluid in the tissues within the body.

Dermoid Cyst: Also known as a cystic teratoma which can occur in the ovary. Dermoid cysts can occur in both females and males in just about any part of the body. Fatty glands, hair, cartilage, bone structures, and teeth can enclose the dermoid cyst within a dermis-type tissue.

Diabetes Insipidus: A rare condition in which the kidneys cannot retain water causing extreme thirst and high urination.

Diabetes Mellitus: A disease of the pancreas that is a metabolic disorder. Insulin production is inhibited in the pancreatic islets or the islets of Langerhans resulting in improper digestion of carbohydrates. The disease can lead to coma and death if untreated.

Dilatation: Type of heart enlargement brought on by congestive heart failure. There is a difference between this condition and cardiac hypertrophy. Dilatation is a pathological condition that happens when the heart muscle fibers stretch to cause an enlargement of the heart or chambers in the heart. The chamber overfills with blood and stretches. Hypertrophy: The normal enlargement of the heart from athletic training. Unlike the athletically enlarged heart, the pathological heart's capillary beds do not increase in size when the heart muscle increases and heart organ oxygen starvation will occur.

Diminished Circulation: Occurs when the embalming fluid does not flow evenly. Copious amounts may be required to plumb emaciated tissues. Sectional embalming may be required along with gentle massage in a slow process for better distribution of fluids. Alternating flooding with drainage will enhance the diffusion of fluids when diminished circulation occurs.

Disease of the Pituitary Gland: Any acromegaly or excessive growth of extremities and head bones which can cause gigantism, dwarfism, diabetes insipidus, hyperthyroidism (which affects women 7 times more often than men), Grave's Disease, and goiter.

Diverticulitis: Refers to when abnormal sacs develop in the colon. Waste accumulates in the sacs and festers causing the diverticula to become inflamed. This inflammation can lead to perforation which can lead to peritonitis.

Dropsy: An edema that describes a local condition in which tissue contains excess fluid. The cause of this edema is due to the boost in permeability of the capillaries. This increased capillary pressure can be induced by venous obstruction or heart failure, inflammation, or other problems associated with body fluids or electrolyte balances.

Dysplasia: Tissue generation which is abnormal in a body.

Dystrophy: Poor nutrition in a body.

Ecchymosis: A bruise which may be the result of a prolonged use of anti-inflammatory drugs. This type of bruise is most often seen in the hands and arms of the deceased. Intravenous drugs and fluids administered before death prevents the removal of these extravascular stains with embalming fluids.

Ectopic Pregnancy: Occurs when the fertilized egg implants itself anywhere that is not the womb or the uterus. An ectopic implantation can be located in the abdominal, cervical, intramural, ovarian, intraligamentous, fimbrial, ampullar, infundibular, isthmic and interstitial tissues. However, the most common mis-implant is in the fallopian tube. The pregnancy hardly ever goes full term due to the fact that the fallopian tube has a risk of blockage or it fails to eject the egg into the uterus. Scarring, previous inflammation, or tubal infections can prevent the egg from properly dropping into the uterus. Sometimes an ectopic pregnancy is idiopathic.

Edema: this term refers to the accumulation of fluid in tissues and accompanying swelling in the body.

Emaciation: Severe weight loss to the point of wasting away from illness or disease.

Embolism: A debris obstruction of a blood vessel. The obstruction is called an embolus. The types of obstructions are blood clots, plaque caused by cholesterol, bacteria, cancer, and fat from the marrow of broken bones, amniotic fluid, or air bubbles.

Encephalitis: Refers to a brain inflammation that is caused by a virus. Primary encephalitis is when a virus infects the brain and spinal cord first. Secondary encephalitis is when a virus infects a different part of the body and then spreads to the spinal cord and brain. Another name for this is post infectious encephalitis. The viruses which cause it are herpes virus, arbovirus and childhood infections.

Endocarditis: That which affects the endocardium (inner lining of the heart); may include the valves or cardiac septum; caused by blood clots that damage/traumatize tissues; bacteria then infects the damaged tissue; can occur after transplanting of artificial heart or IV drugs; can spread to kidneys or renal blood vessel linings.

Endometriomas: Occurs when the egg cells get into the ovary rather than the uterus. These cells collect blood causing ovarian blood cysts. These cysts can grow to the size of an orange and be very painful to the female.

Endometriosis: A condition which causes painful menstrual cycles, pain during or after sexual intercourse, painful bowel movements and can cause infertility. The endometrium or the lining of the uterus tissue grows in other areas of the abdomen than in the uterus. The tissue is programmed to detach itself from the uterus each month and slough off through the menstrual cycle. Tissue in other areas cannot detach itself and this causes cramps and pain during the cycle each month. This may inhibit the egg from proceeding through the fallopian tube to the uterus. It can cause scarring and tissue damage to the tube, the ovaries, fallopian tubes and other areas.

Enteritis: Inflammation of the lining of the intestines within the body. This is caused by microorganisms in the stomach and intestines which inflame the intestines. Staphylococcus, Salmonella, Shigella, Campylobacter and E. coli are some of the microbes which cause enteritis.

Entry of pathogens: The parts of the body that pathogens use to gain entry into the body. Skin is invaded through sores, cuts, or abrasions. The mucous membranes in nose, eyes, and ears are infected from rubbing infected hands or objects. The respiratory tract is invaded by airborne microbes. The digestive tract is contaminated by food and drink ingestion. The genitourinary tract can be contaminated and spread infections in the urinary and reproductive organs. The placenta is vulnerable during pregnancy. Pregnant embalmers can pass cytomegalovirus, CMV, through the placenta wall to their fetus.

Epistaxis: A nose bleed which comes from the nasal septum when a dilated blood vessel is harmed. An epistaxis can also be caused from cancer or blood clot.

Erythrocytosis: A condition in which red blood cells increase.

Esophagitis: Inflammation of the esophagus which is caused by reflux of bile into the esophagus.

Etiology: The study of the causes of disease.

Exit of pathogens: Refers to the body fluids: secretions and blood, feces, urine, semen, sputum, saliva, blood, pus, tears and vaginal secretions.

Exotoxin: Chemical secretion which is a protein soluble in the surrounding fluid. Some microbes are considered more virulent because of the exotoxins released by them and are more damaging to human tissue than others.

Exsanguination: Excessive bleeding from anywhere on the body which can result in death. The literal meaning of the word is "to drain of blood." Sudden, accidental detachment of a limb, a ruptured aneurysm, or a gunshot can cause this kind of bleeding.

Febrile: A feverish condition.

Fibrillation: Occurrence of the weakened heart cells quivering or spontaneously contracting.

Fibrinolysin: The digestion of fibrin threads.

Focal Infections: Infections that result in pneumonia, tonsillitis, septic arthritis, osteomyelitis, peritonitis, and/or meningitis.

Fomite: An inanimate object on which an infectious pathogen clings as on a table surface.

Fractures: Broken bones. There are two types categorized by compound or bone which protrudes through the skin and simple where no protrusion of bone occurs.

Functional Cyst: Refers to when a follicle forms but does not burst to release the egg. Fluid will collect in it and then in 60 days it will disappear. Benign or malignant cysts are different and must be treated accordingly.

Furuncle: A boil on the skin.

Gangrene: Necrosis combined with decomposition.

Gastritis: Inflammation of the stomach within the body. Gastritis is caused by extreme alcohol consumption, some drugs, ulcer-causing bacteria, pernicious anemia, and autoimmune disorders

Gastrointestinal Infections: Digestive diseases which are caused by bacteria, viruses or fungus.

Gingivitis: Inflammation of the gums in the mouth. Gingivitis is caused by plaque build-up on the teeth next to the gums. Plaque consists of food particles, mucous and bacteria and hardens into tartar. Gingivitis is common in person's suffering from diabetes, hormonal changes with pregnancy and poor dental hygiene.

Glomerulonephritis: A microbiological disorder caused by inflammation of the glomerulus and the nephron. This is the most acute and debilitating renal disorder.

Goiter: Abnormal growth of the thyroid gland from a lack of iodine.

Hematemesis: Vomiting of blood. Some common causes are due to ulcers in the upper gastrointestinal tract or stomach and esophagus inflammation.

Hematin: A chemical component that is black.

Hematuria: Blood in the urine. The blood usually originates from the urethra, bladder, ureters, kidneys or prostate gland. This can be determined either microscopically or by gross investigation. Gross means that a visible indicator can be viewed. One visible indicator is when urine turns pink, red or brown and has clots. Causes can range from kidney stones/diseases, medications, trauma, tumors, infections, STDs, Sickle Cell Anemia, systemic lupus erythematosus and prostate enlargement.

Hemolytic Anemia: The rupturing of red blood cells caused by a congenital disorder or toxic agents. The hemoglobin breaks down into heme and globin thus reducing the amount of oxygen-carrying hemoglobin in the system. Pernicious Anemia: this term refers to the intestine's inability to produce chemicals that helps absorb vitamin B12. This helps the body absorb iron. Iron is the main part of heme that is half of hemoglobin which carries oxygen.

Hemolytic Disease: Present in a newborn that is due to Rh factor. The antibodies of the Rh negative mother cross the placenta to create the Rh positive factor in the infant.

Hemophilia: Hereditary condition in which sometimes excessive bleeding and spontaneous bleeding occurs. Type A and B Hemophilia are characterized by low to zero levels of the protein which causes the blood to clot. Administering blood clotting factors usually solve this disorder.

Hemoptysis: The expulsion of bloody spittle from the respiratory tract.

Hemorrhage: Any interior or exterior leaking of blood from the vascular system that has been caused by trauma, disease, or high blood pressure.

Hemorrhoids: Inflammation of the rectum blood vessels in the body.

Hepatitis: Inflammation of the liver. Parasites, bacteria, viruses, illicit drug use, and alcohol in combination with acetaminophen are all causes of this disease. Autoimmune hepatitis is another form of this disease. Cystic fibrosis or excess copper in the body also leads to this disease. Risk factors for contracting the disease include: contaminated foods, unprotected sex, drug abuse, living in a nursing home, extreme alcohol consumption, organ transplant, AIDS, getting a tattoo, health care or funeral home workers. Jaundice, or yellow tint of skin, mucous membranes and eyes is a red flag to embalmers that there are potentially numerous varieties of microbes present causing hepatitis.

Hyaluronidase: The enzymes produced which cause acute damage. This causes the blood to clot which produces fibrin threads in the blood stream.

Hydrocele: Edema of the scrotum.

Hydropericardium: Excess fluid in the pericardial sac which surrounds the heart of the body.

Hydrothorax: Excessive fluid in the thoracic cavity or in the pleural cavity which can cause purge if the fluid is not aspirated along with any hemorrhage. Proper preparation of the chest cavity will reduce microbe growth which can also cause purge. Universal precautions must be taken or the embalmer runs the risk of infections from any respiratory maladies suffered by the decedent.

Hyperemia: Increased blood flow to a particular area of the body.

Hypertension: Refers to high blood pressure. High blood pressure is mostly idiopathic in nature. Hypertensive heart disease stems from hypertension (high blood pressure). When the left ventricle hypertrophies (enlarges pathologically), its requirement for more nutrients increases but the heart cannot produce more because it is enlarged. The left ventricle wall's enlargement also causes it to pump less efficiently which reduces blood output.

Hypoxia: Decrease in the level of oxygen in the tissue.

Impetigo: The streptococcal infection that is located in the skin and underlying tissues.

Inclusion: Any material in an organ, cell, or tissue which is of a foreign nature and not caused by injury.

Inflammation: A condition of swelling, fever, redness, joint aches, muscle pains, exhaustion and organ dysfunction or altered function. A person experiencing inflammatory symptoms is a person with an immune system that is working to restrain and eradicate damage within the cell. An injured cell will be attacked by foreign organisms. This process removes dead cells and tissues that have been injured. If the tissue cannot be repaired, then the inflammation process forms scar tissue to replace necrotic tissue in the cell.

Insufficiency: A congenital condition where the valves of the heart do not perform properly.

Irreversible Stage: A critical point in which no amount of medical help can revive the body's functionality. The damage to vital body tissues such as the cardiac muscle cannot be repaired.

Ischemia: Decrease or reduction of blood flow to an organ. Fainting is caused by mildly restricted blood flow to the brain, whereas stroke is caused by a severe restriction of blood flow to the brain.

Ischemic Stroke: Also abbreviated as TIA. This occurs when a blood vessel is blocked and deprives brain tissue of blood. The result causes symptoms which last for a short time from an hour to a day.

Jaundice: Yellowing of skin commonly found on someone who has died of liver dysfunction.

Leucopenia: A change in blood composition with decreased white blood cells. Causes of this disease are found in the failure of bone marrow to produce white blood cells, HIV, as well as a variety of chemical agents. This is a common condition after radiation or chemotherapy.

Leukemia: White blood cell cancer or cancer of the tissues that synthesize white blood cells. Four forms of it are myelocytic (AML), acute lymphocytic (ALL), chronic myeloid (CML) and chronic lymphocytic (CLL). This is a hematopoietic disorder.

Leukocytosis: A disease where there is an increase in white blood cells. It is not leukemia which is a white blood cell cancer. Causes of this disease are found in the changes in the blood such as hemorrhage, extensive surgeries, coronary occlusions, cancer, pregnancy, chemical intoxication, and toxemias.

Leukopenia: A white blood cell count decrease or reduction.

Lipase: Enzyme which acts with oil and fats to allow Staphylococcus to live in the skin.

Lumpectomy: A lump that is removed. The lump is a mass or tumor.

Malignant: Cancerous tumor. Cancer is derived from the Latin word for crab because cancer spreads out into surrounding tissues in the shape of a crab. This spread is called metastasis. Malignant tumors infiltrate and can reoccur after removal. These tumors can cause extensive damage that can alter the body. These changes are fatal if not treated.

Mallory-Weiss Tears: Caused by the violent retching of an alcoholic resulting in a tear in the esophageal varices which causes massive bleeding and death.

Mastectomy: Removal of the breast because it is too full of diseased tissue to save. This operation entails the removal of the whole breast or a section of the breast. There are 4 types: Subcutaneous is the removal of breast without the removal of the nipple and areola. Total means that all that was left is the axillary lymph nodes. The modified radical leaves most of the axillary lymph nodes. A radical is the removal of breast, muscles and all lymph nodes, but this method is in rarely used by modern doctors.

Mechanical Transmission: Occurs when the insect carries the pathogen from the source and deposits the pathogen on the potential host as when a fly goes to feces and then lands on food contaminating it.

Melena: Black or tarry feces common in newborns. This occurs because of the digestion of blood in the upper digestive tract due to the fact that the digestion of blood takes a longer period of time to be broken down into hematin. Ulcers or gastritis can lead to this condition.

Meningitis: Occurs from two microbes, Streptococcus pneumoniae and Neisseria meningitides. It is contagious and is an infection of the cerebrospinal fluid.

Metastasis: A cancer that spreads all over the body and which can cause blockage from tumor cells which break off a tumor and lodge in a smaller vein blocking blood flow causing an embolism.

Microbes: Microscopic organisms which secrete chemicals that are toxic to the human system.

Morbidity Rate: The number of sick people to well people in a given population.

Mortality Rate: The number of deaths to the total population.

Multiple Sclerosis: A central nervous system inflammation. It is an autoimmune disorder and is thought to be linked to a viral infection. It invades the lymphocytes. Lymphocytes are the T cells and macrophages. The disorder degrades the myelin sheath of the nerves.

Myelitis: Inflammation of the spinal cord which causes an infection and necrosis of the spinal cord or demyelization of the spinal cord which is called transverse myelitis. There is no treatment or cure for it and it results in a serious disability.

Myocardial Infarction: Refers to MI or a heart attack. An obstruction in the artery supplying a certain area causes necrosis in the tissue. Drainage of the area becomes blocked, although thrombosis in the artery that brings blood into the heart is more common. Angina pectoris is the chest pain that comes with the MI. The pain may occur for several days or weeks before the MI occurs. When the MI occurs, the pain increases with exertion, eating a big meal or exposure to cold. Symptoms: crushing pressure behind breastbone; chest pain that spreads out to neck, jaw, abdomen, shoulder, or left arm; nausea, vomiting, difficulty breathing, anxiety or fear. This pain is not affected by coughing, deep breathing or swallowing.

Neoplasm: A tumor. Oncologists study tumors in a science called oncology. This term originates from the word neoplasia which means "new growth".

Nephrolithiasis: The condition in which kidney stones are formed.

Non-obstructed Atelectasis: Can be caused by various conditions including congestive heart failure, blood or air within the pleural cavity, lack of contact between parietal and visceral pleurae, lack of surfactant, scarring and even compression. Air becomes trapped between the outside and the inside of the lung, and the lung is prevented from contracting and expanding due to the even pressure. Finally, the lung collapses because it cannot fully expand.

Nosocomial: Infections that originate from treatment gained in a hospital or health care clinic.

Obstructed Atelectasis: This condition occurs when the trachea or the bronchi becomes blocked by food or other obstructions. Tumors or fungal infections in the respiratory system and extreme amounts of mucous collecting in the throat or airways can also cause blockage. Mucous blocking diseases include asthma, bronchitis, cystic fibrosis, paralysis and amyotrophic lateral sclerosis.

Oliguria: A reduction in the production of urine.

Orchitis: Testes inflammation injury, metastasis, or infection in the body of a person.

Osmotic Pressure: Pressure between two solutions of differing concentrations that is separated by a semi-permeable membrane on the cellular level.

Osteoarthritis: A type of arthritis which is degenerative cartilage.

Osteomalacia: An adult disease which leads to a softening of the bones caused by deficient calcification.

Osteomyelitis: Inflamed bones and bone marrow caused by bacteria.

Osteoporosis: this term refers to a loss of bone mass. The condition creates fragile bones prone to fractures and breaking.

Osteosarcoma: Most common type of bone cancer.

Ovarian cysts: Fluid-filled sacs that form on or in the ovaries. Usually they will form and then disappear without treatment.

Pancreatitis: Inflammation of the pancreas in the body. It is caused by its own enzymes digesting it due to blockage of the duct and the pancreatic juices which begin digesting in the pancreas. This is called autolysis or a self-digestion of tissues.

Paralysis: A nerve disorder which can atrophy muscles and diminishes circulation.

Parkinson's disease: this term refers to a disorder which has symptoms and possible treatments documented as early as 5000 B.C. It is the brain disorder in which there is a lack of the messenger chemical dopamine which controls muscle movement. It affects muscles, facial movements, walk, posture and strength. It is idiopathic.

Passive hyperemia: When blood does not drain properly from an organ, but venous blood keeps coming into the organ. This condition is associated with heart failure and produces a reddish-blue hue to the body part. The hue deepens as the blood loses oxygen. This discoloration is cyanosis.

Pathogenesis: The beginning of a lesion formation.

Peptic ulcers: Wearing away of the lining of the stomach or duodenum of the small intestine. The dead tissue is cast off and that leaves a hole which food particles and bacteria can enter the abdominal cavity.

Pericarditis: Inflammation of area between outside of the heart and pericardium (protective sac around the heart); causes - blunt force trauma, infection. Cardiac Tamponade: Excessive fluid collects in the inflamed areas; fluid disturbs the balance of electrolyte and protein within the sac, causes pressure against the heart; prevents the heart from fully contracting or expanding, causing a drop in blood pressure, which causes more accumulation of fluid.

Peritonitis: Inflammation of the membrane surrounding the abdominal cavity. Peritonitis can be a fatal condition.

Petechiae: Tiny hemorrhages of capillaries or mucous membranes just under the skin. The appearance is flat, round spots with colors ranging in red to purple. Embalming fluids do not remove the petechiae due to the fact that the fluids cause an extravascular stain.

Phagocytes: (Neutrophils, monocytes, and macrophages) surround and obliterate the rubble and foreign matter and remove them from the wound.

Phagocytosis: Refers to how the white blood cells work to destroy the micro-foreigners.

Pharyngitis: Inflammation of the pharynx which is symptomatic of a sore throat. Pharyngitis is caused by microbes, mostly viruses, the same viruses that cause colds, flu, HIV, and other illnesses. Bacterial causes consist of streptococcus, Corynebacterium, Neisseria gonorrhoeae and Chlamydia pneumoniae. The embalmer should be aware of these potential hazards when inflammation is present in the deceased.

Phlebitis: Inflammation of leg veins which causes blood clots that can reduce mobility. It can also lead to blood pooling or blood clotting.

Pitting Edema: An excess of fluid in the arms and legs of the body. This condition is indicated by pressing a finger against the skin to see if the skin retains the finger depression.

Plaque: The cholesterol, cellular waste, calcium or other fragmentation of substances that can clog the arteries.

Pleurisy: The pleurae and occurs when the pleural is infected with microorganisms. Forming pus can cause empyema. Fibrous substance may stick to the diaphragm or chest wall in this disorder of the lower respiratory tract.

Pneumoconiosis: Caused by inhaling mineral dust such as coal (black lung or anthracosis), asbestos (Asbestosis), silica (Silicosis), and beryllium (Berylliosis). Dust gets into the respiratory system and most of it is removed by the ciliated epithelial lining of the tract. Macrophages form and the cells release chemicals in an effort to expunge the trapped dust particles. This amalgamation of dust and immune system chemicals are toxic to the lungs. Fibrous material form and can cause emphysema which is air pockets at the ends of the bronchioles. The person can inhale but can't exhale properly: smoking and infections can cause this, too.

Pneumonia: Respiratory disorder which is caused by bacteria and viruses that produces an inflammation of the lungs.

Polycythemia Vera: An idiopathic disorder also known as erythrocytosis which is an unusually high red blood cell count. There is an increase in thickness or viscosity of the blood with high concentrations of hemoglobin. Thrombi and clotting of the blood are the result. Other symptoms include: weakness, fatigue, vertigo, tinnitus, irritability, enlarged spleen, ruddy discoloration of the face, pain and redness in the arms and legs, black and blue spots on the skin, coma and stroke. This is treated with radioactive phosphorus 32P which can be dangerous to the embalmer.

Primary anemia: Decreased production of red blood cells in the body.

Prognosis: The probable development of a disease and its outcome by a physician.

Progressive Stage: Condition that worsens after the compensatory devices of the body fail to oxygenate the body tissues. This condition worsens until shock reaches the next stage or medical help arrives to help the body regulate sufficient blood flow.

Prolapse: Occurs when the valve is stretched out of shape preventing it from closing properly.

Psoriatic: A type of arthritis that is a chronic condition associated with psoriasis affecting the fingers and toes.

Pulmonary Edema: Collection of fluid in the lungs which can be a life threatening condition due to the restrictions on the oxygen and carbon dioxide exchange.

Purge: Any blood appearing in the nose, mouth or ears. Purge from the lungs is frothy red or black like coffee grounds. Purge from the stomach is pink. Purge from the brain is clear. The embalmer must treat the cause of the purge to prevent its possible reoccurrence during the funeral or viewing. Purge can be caused by gas build up or edema in the brain.

Purpura: Spontaneous bleeding in the tissues which leaves discolorations of red or purple in the skin. This usually disappears after a few weeks. In the decedent, the discoloration is permanent and cannot be removed by embalming fluid.

Pustule: A small elevation of the skin.

Pyelitis: Renal pelvis and calyx's kidney inflammation. Both can be caused from microbes which migrate from the bladder to the kidneys.

Pyelonephritis: Inflammation of the basic structure and functional units of the kidneys or nephrons caused by renal infections.

Rapid coagulation of blood: Lack of fluid which can lead to rapid blood clotting as well as liver damage.

Rapid Decomposition: this term refers to excess fluid and high body temperatures which increase the rate of decomposition.

Reactive Arthritis: Formerly known as Reiter's Syndrome which attacks the cartilage of joints. Salmonella is one, but not the only, bacterium which induces this type of arthritis.

Regeneration: Damaged cells replaced by same type of cells as the affected tissue and returns the tissue to normal.

Remission: Abatement of a disease or the symptoms of a disease.

Resolution: Refers to what happens when the affected tissue is returned to a normal state or condition.

Restoration: Damaged tissue replaced by cells not necessarily of same type as the affected tissue and returns the tissue to normal.

Rheumatic Heart Disease: A bacterial infection from strep throat. Rheumatic fever bacteria may lay dormant for years before injuring the mitral valve. In most cases, it can lead to endocarditis and infection of multiple layers of the heart and can lead to cardiac failure.

Rheumatoid: A type of arthritis which is an inflammation of the joint linings or organs.

Rhinitis: Upper respiratory tract and is exhibited by inflamed nasal passages.

Rickets: A disease which occurs in infants and children caused by a deficiency of vitamin D and causing defective bone growth. Poor levels of calcium and phosphate contribute to the softening of bones.

Ruptured Aneurysm: A blood-filled sac dilation of an artery. This can cause excessive bleeding and lead to death.

Salmonella bacteria: Bacteria which can cause nausea, vomiting, diarrhea, cramps, and fever within 6 to 72 hours of contamination exposure. The bacterium is ingested from infected food or drink, or can be passed from an infected person to healthy persons.

Salpingitis: Fallopian tube (female) or Eustachian tube inflammation.

Scar Formation: Cicatrix or the repaired tissue of connecting tissues.

Scoliosis: Spinal curvature in the back.

Sebaceous Cyst: A cheese-like material filled sac just under the skin. This sac is also known as an epidermal cyst, keratin cyst, or epidermoid cyst and results from swollen hair follicles or trauma to the skin. They can return after being surgically removed, but are usually painless. Some have been known to become inflamed and painful.

Secondary Anemia: The loss or destruction of red blood cells in the body.

Sickle Cell Anemia: A person with this disease has sickle shaped red blood cells which is the physical effect of the abnormal hemoglobin molecule. It is inherited only when both parents have the recessive hemoglobin S gene. The damaged bone marrow is extremely painful. Fat emboli can spread from the dead tissue of the bone marrow and cause sudden death through stroke or heart failure. Persons of African or Mediterranean ancestry are predominantly affected. It can lead to other severe conditions: anemia, heart problems, damage to kidneys, joints and muscles, brain, lungs, spleen. These result in tower skull, physical fatigue, heart failure, kidney failure, arthritis, paralysis, pneumonia, and/or spleen fibrosis.

Sinusitis: Upper respiratory tract and is exhibited in the inflammation of sinus cavities. It could be one or all four of the cavities which are connected to the nasal passages. Rhinitis and sinusitis are two conditions that can be caused by chemical irritants, infections or allergies.

Staphylococcal Infections: Bacteria that can cause the spread of communicable infections. Staph infections are caused by bacteria which generally are associated with forming abscesses and are the leading cause of nosocomial infections. Staph exists on the skin or in the nostrils of about 20% of humans. It is found in the mouth, breast tissue, genitals, urinary and upper respiratory tracts. Staphylococcal aureus is common and found on 70%-90% of the earth's population, although 40% never develop any symptoms. Staph is exhibited in a ring of bacteria and dead white blood cells or abscesses on the skin or deep in tissue. It causes boils, impetigo, Toxic Shock Syndrome (TSS) and staphylococcal scalded skin syndrome (SSSS).

Stenosis: An acquired defect in which the valve opening narrows and restricts the blood flow.

Stoma: Opening in the neck that indicates a tracheotomy or a laryngectomy was performed. This may complicate arterial injection of the embalming fluids. The stoma should be removed and the opening sutured after proper disinfecting and packing of the opening.

Strep Throat: The streptococcal infection that is located in the pharynx. Scarlet Fever: this term refers to the streptococcal infection that is located in the upper body of the person.

Streptococcus pyogenes: Bacteria known as GAS or S. pyogenes which causes the streptococcal infections. These bacteria are in Group A and are penicillin sensitive. A carbohydrate capsule surrounds the bacterium to protect it from attack by the macrophages or immune antibodies. The M protein prohibits the immune system from attaching to the bacteria and destroying it. The M protein is what the antibodies use to identify the bacterium and is the weakest link. GAS releases toxins and enzymes for spreading infection and digesting the protein in blood clotting. Types of disease are usually known by the location of the infection.

Thrombocytopenia: A reduction in platelet count and can cause several bleeding disorders.

Thrombosis: Blood clot formation that is stationary, but has the potential to disintegrate into the blood stream. It can be caused by injury to the blood vessel, a slowing of blood flow, a change in blood make-up, a disease of the blood or genetic mutation. Endothelial lining damage causes thrombocytes to accumulate on a spot in the lining of the blood vessel. This type of clot is usually in the heart or arteries. The end result can be death.

Tracheitis: A disorder of the upper respiratory tract which affects the trachea and is usually caused by biological infection, most often the bacteria Staphylococcus aureus. This is accompanied by a blockage of the trachea and affects young children more than adults. Sometimes it requires insertion of a tube for breathing called an endotracheal tube.

Tuberculosis: A communicable disease that has become multi-drug resistant in several forms. Mycobacterium tuberculosis is the bacteria which are spread by a cough or sneeze in the air. The World Health Organization has designated a world emergency from this disease on a worldwide level. The danger in the bacteria is its survivor type, which can last for long periods in dried blood or spittle. It causes cavitation which is basically cavities in the lung tissue or other organs affected by the disease.

Typhoid Fever: Enteric fever which is caused by Salmonella typhi bacteria. Transmission of this disease is most frequently from poor hygiene and public sanitation practices. The feces of an infected person can contaminate water or food which is transferred to a person who ingests the food or water.

Ulcer: An open sore or mucus membrane that sloughs off inflamed necrotic tissues.

Ulcerative Colitis: Refers to the large intestines and rectum that is characterized by ulcers. It is a bowel inflammation in which the epithelial cells have been killed in the lining of the colon. It is idiopathic. Up to 40% of patients must have all or portions of their colon removed due to excessive bleeding or cancer risk. Sometimes, a colostomy is performed where a hole in the abdomen is made. This is called a stoma and waste is excreted through this hole.

Ureteritis: Inflammation of one or both the ureters. Urethritis is the inflamed urethra tube which carries urine out of the body. It is caused by microbes traveling from the vagina and the anus to the urethra. Venereal diseases are the main infectious agents indicated by yellow-green pus in the urethra.

Valvular Defects: The valves that keep the blood flowing in the direction it should flow. The three basic ways that valves disrupt this flow are, insufficiency, stenosis and prolapse. The tricuspid valve and pulmonic valve may become diseased. The more common defects are in the aortic and mitral valves. Deformed valves are prone to infection. Valvular defects and blood vessel disorders restrict the proper flow of embalming fluid to all parts of the body. Blood clots, increased blood viscosity, weakened or ruptured blood vessels are the bane of embalmers. Use of pre-injection and co-injection chemicals induce chemical changes which help proper flow of the embalming fluids.

Varicose Veins: Enlarged veins close to the skin's surface in the lower extremities which is caused by excessive blood pressure.

Vasoconstriction: Refers to how the tiny veins around the trauma constrict for 15-30 minutes to keeps any toxins or foreign organisms from spreading.

Vasodilatation: Histamine-like chemicals released to cause the veins to dilate and wash away the toxins or foreigners from the wound. Redness, swelling and heat occur at the wound site.

Venereal Diseases: Sexually transmitted diseases or STDs. There is a difference between sexually transmitted disease and sexually transmitted infections or STIs. STDs are caused by germs like viruses, bacteria or parasites. The body exhibits the symptoms of these infectious agents. STI means that a person can be carrying the germs and can transmit the germs. Persons with STIs do not necessarily show symptoms of infection. STIs are transmitted through mucous membranes of the penis, vulva, and mouth. Bacteria, fungi, protozoa, or viruses cause the infection, not the sexual activity.

Vesicle: A blister or a sac on top of the skin filled with fluid.

Zoonoses: The transmission of zoonotic disease by animals or insects.

Zoonotic Disease: Diseases such as rabies or malaria which are carried by animals or insects.

Chemistry

Divisions and definition

Chemistry is the study of the nature of matter and the changes, alterations, or transformation that occurs in matter. The main divisions of chemistry include: inorganic chemistry, organic chemistry, biochemistry, and embalming chemistry. Inorganic chemistry is the study of minerals found on earth. These minerals are found in compounds, molecules, atoms, crystals and metals. Organic chemistry is the study of carbon compounds. Biochemistry studies the living organism. These living organisms can be found in certain types of compounds or reactions which occur. The embalming chemistry is the study of disinfection and the preservation of human remains. The study includes the matter and the changes that occur in the process of embalming. Chemistry has many other subdivisions. These include Analytical Chemistry, Nuclear Chemistry, Physical Chemistry, and a number of specialized studies. The exact nature of this experimental science requires careful attention to detail by the scientist.

Metric System

The International System of Units (SI) or the Metric System allows a standard set of measurement and was initiated in 1960. The embalmer uses: length, volume, mass and heat. The exact standard based on incremental graduations of 10 should be applied in this experimental science to ensure the proper results. Length is measured in meters, but can be subdivided into divisions of decimeter, centimeter, millimeter, and micron or multiplied to form kilometer. Volume is measured as 1 meter cubed. Labs use the decimeter (1/10) or liter. Mass = gram with 1000 grams equaling a kilogram and 1 gram equaling 1000 mg. Weight changes with the distance from gravity center whereas mass is the quantity of matter present in the object. Heat = calorie and is measured by the quantity necessary to raise the temperature of 1 gram of water by 1° Celsius at 15° Celsius.

Exothermic and endothermic

Solid, liquid, gas are the three states of matter. The amount of energy it possesses determines the state of any substance. Heat is a form of energy. When heat is liberated, then the substance will turn from a gas to solid state and when heat is absorbed, the substance will turn from a solid state to a gaseous state. This is illustrated by the formation of ice, heat is liberated and a solid is formed. When the ice melts, heat is absorbed and the ice melts. When even more heat is absorbed, then steam forms. **Exothermic** is the liberation or releasing of heat that allows a gas to turn into a liquid state and in turn that form will turn to a solid state. **Endothermic** is the absorbing of heat that allows a solid to turn into a liquid and liquid to form into gas.

Atoms and valence

An atom refers to the smallest particle of a chemical element which still retains the properties of that element. The composition includes smaller particles: neutron, proton and electron. The number of the subatomic particles determines the element of the atom. A valence is the formed by atoms. The valence is the number of chemical bonds an element has which are formed by atoms. Valence electrons are those in the outermost energy level and these determine the chemical properties of the atom. The importance regarding this number of valence electrons can be found in looking at the atoms which have the same number of electrons. These atoms typically have the same chemical and physical properties as their counterparts. Electrons travel in energy levels and so like electrons stick together. The lower the level number, the closer to the nucleus. The closer to the nucleus, the fewer electrons in orbit. The farther away from the nucleus, the more electrons in orbit.

Chemical reactions

Chemical reactions are the result of substances in the process of interconversion. Reactants are the substances which act in response to each other. For example, an acid and a metal cause a chemical reaction. Reactants form or break chemical bonds producing a chemical change in the substances. This results in a product different than either substance which originally created it. In the example acid and metal, a corrosive substance is produced. This process involves the exchanging of electrons which are usually the valence electrons which determine the chemical property of the substance. Electrons are charged with negative electricity. Reactions are subdivided into organic reactions and inorganic reactions. Organic reactions involve carbon-based substances. Inorganic reactions are those which involve compounds that are not carbon. The carbon connections are formed from minerals, salts, acids, oxides and carbides. The branch of organic chemistry that deals with life processes is known as biochemistry.

Saponification in corpses

Saponification is also known as adipocere. Adipocere has a more common name which is grave wax. This process is the conversion of a high fat content tissue into a soap-like substance. The soap-like substance is resistant to bacterial growth and decomposition. This substance starts to form approximately one month after the burial of the body. However, the substance can remain for centuries within the body. This substance is produced from a hydrolysis process. Hydrolysis is a chemical process in which a fatty molecule reacts with a water (H_2O) molecule. The fatty molecule is split apart and one part receives an OH from the water molecule and the other receives an H^+ from the water molecule. A different substance unlike fat or water is produced. This process usually occurs in wet ground or under water that has a high alkaline content. However, an exposed body is unlikely to undergo this adipocerous process.

Arrhenius, Brønsted-Lowery and Lewis

Arrhenius is an acid-base chemical reaction. The formula ($2H2O \rightleftarrows H3O+ + OH-$) is descriptive of Svante Arrhenius definition of this term. He went on to further characterize acid as a compound causing an increase in H3O+ and a decrease in OH-. The compound which causes the reverse reaction is a base. Arrhenius is a substance which yields hydrogen or hydronium ions in water. **Bronsted-Lowry** is a substance developed by Johann Nicolas Bronsted and Martin Lowery in 1923, hence its name. This substance has an acid's capability *to donate a proton* H^+ to a base. This substance can account for the reactions outside a solution, unlike the substance Arrhenius which does not have this capability. **Lewis** has the reactivity of an acid and is described by its ability to *accept a pair of electrons* from a base. The base is characterized as an electron-pair donor. This reaction forms a covalent bond. Covalent bonds are intermolecular chemical bonds with one or more pairs of shared electrons. The covalent bond is directional caused by the form of the orbitals (s, p, d, f) or hybrid orbitals.

Required knowledge

The embalmer must have a solid understanding of the principles relating to organic chemistry, inorganic chemistry and biochemistry. A foundation of knowledge concerning the basic chemical principles enables the embalmer to select the correct chemicals used in the embalming process. The use of chemicals in the mortuary and crematory are essential. Potential hazards of the chemicals can occur if the embalmer is not fully aware of the regulations concerning hazardous chemicals. The embalmer should be able to formulate the embalming fluid in appropriate strengths and select them based on the condition of the decedent. The embalmer should be able to use appropriate applications of disinfectants and other topical chemicals in the preparation of the body. Hypodermic treatments may also be needed. Be able to understand and recognize illnesses, treatments, and the effects of medication that could cause potential harmful interactions with embalming fluids.

Laws of Conservation

The **Law of the Conservation of Energy** holds that no chemical or physical change can destroy mass. In exchanging the word mass for the word energy, energy is depicted as an inflow of energy that must equal the outflow of energy. This allows that energy could change from one form of energy into another form of energy. Energy that existed is never created or destroyed, but transformed into another state of being. This concept is based upon the idea that the total energy in a closed system will remain constant. The **Law of Conservation of Mass** is consistent in remaining constant or stable in a closed system. The mass of the reactants will equal or amount to equal mass of the product in any chemical process. This law is used in many industries including fluid dynamics.

Formula subscript number calculations

The proper way to view a subscript number in H_2O is to see that the 2 is indicative that there are two atoms of hydrogen and one atom of oxygen present. When two atoms are acting as one unit such as the OH group then the proper way to use a subscript is to put the unit in parentheses $(OH)_2$ which indicates there are 2 oxygen atoms, and 2 hydrogen atoms, but the oxygen/hydrogen atoms are acting as one unit. Compounds such as calcium bicarbonate are written $Ca(HCO_3)_2$ The compound (HCO_3) has one hydrogen atom, one carbon atom, and three oxygen atoms. In $Ca(HCO_3)_2$ you should see that there are two hydrogen atoms, two carbon atoms, and 6 oxygen atoms. In $2Ca(HCO_3)_2$, you see 2 calcium atoms, 4 hydrogen atoms, 4 carbon atoms, 12 oxygen atoms, and 2 calcium bicarbonate molecules.

Atomic structure of elements

The atomic structure of elements determines the chemical combination and the proportion by mass of a compound. Compounds which exist in a stable state have 2 electrons in the outer orbit or 8 electrons in the outer orbit. Reaching this state makes an element stable. However, to reach this stability an element must either give up or acquire electrons. There are three ways to describe the bonding that takes place in an element. Chemical bonds are ionic, covalent, or polar covalent. Ionic bonds occur when two electrons are transferred from one atom to another. Covalent bonds occur when the electrons are shared between like atoms. Polar covalent is the most common and occurs in the atom which experiences the most electronegativity. Atoms with the most electronegativity experience more from the electron than the nucleus of the electropositive atoms.

Important terms

Alcohol: Any organic compound where a hydroxyl (-OH) group is bound to a carbon atom of an alkyl. The general formula is R-OH. R describes the hydrocarbon group. An alkyl is a univalent radical with only carbon and hydrogen combined in a chain.

Aldehyde: An organic compound where a carbon atom bonded to a hydrogen atom double-bonded to an oxygen atom. The formula is RCHO where R is the hydrocarbon group or hydrogen. An aldehyde group chemical formula is –CHO. It is also called the formyl group. HCHO is formaldehyde.

Aldose: this term refers to a sugar where the functional groups are hydroxyl (-OH) groups and aldehyde (-CHO) groups.

Alkane: A saturated hydrocarbon. The general formula is $CnH(2n + 2)$. This substance is also known as the paraffin series. This substance has the maximum number of hydrogen atoms possible which ensures that it is a hydrocarbon with no double bonds.

Alkene: A type of hydrocarbon that has carbon-carbon double bonds (ethylene).

Alkyl group: A type of monovalent radical. The general formula is $CnH(2n+1)$. This substance is formed when one hydrogen atom is lost from their position in part of a larger molecular chain. If singled out on their own, they are highly reactive free radicals.

Alkyl halide: A type of hydrocarbon which is a non-aromatic organic compound, or aliphatic.

Alkyne: A type of hydrocarbon that has carbon-carbon triple bonds (acetylene).

Allotropism: Term used when an element exists in two or more physical forms or structures.

Amide: A molecule derived from ammonia substitution for hydrogen or acid. The formula from hydrogen: $C=O$. The formula from acid: –N-H2 for the –OH group.

Amine: A compound which contains nitrogen and is formulated from ammonia when an organic radical replaces one or more hydrogen atoms. The formula: R-NH-L.

Amino acid: The foundation molecule found in protein. This molecule consists of an NH2 amino group, COOH carboxyl group, and a radical.

Amphoteric: A molecule which can be either acidic or a base depending upon the medium's pH levels. The pH levels affect the negative or positive charge of the molecule's structure.

Anion: A negatively charged atom which means that it has more electrons than protons.

Aromatic: A substance which has electrons free to cycle around circular-arranged atoms in either a composition that is singly or doubly bonded. Examples of this substance include: benzene or toluene.

Arrhenius Base: Matter which yields or generates hydroxide ions in water.

Atom: The smallest speck of a substance which still holds on and maintains the properties of the original substance.

Autolysis: A system of the body whereby enzymes digest cells in a form of self-destruction.

Biochemistry: The study of living organism compounds in scientific circles.

Boiling: The state in which liquid changes to vapor states or conditions.

Bronsted-Lowry Base: The compound which tends to accept or receive protons.

Buffers: Neutralized acids and bases within a solution. Acids are neutralized when the pH balance is maintained in the fluid and the body.

Calorie: A measurement of heat in which the temperature of 1 gram of water at 15°C is raised or elevated 1°C.

Carbohydrate: A compound which is the elemental make-up of hydrogen, carbon and oxygen and includes sugars, starches and glycogen.

Carboxylic Acid: An organic compound which contains the group COOH.

Catalyst: A chemical compound which maintains its own properties and holds stable, even when it causes chemical reactions in other substances.

Cation: An atom or group of atoms with a positive charge which means that there are more protons than electrons.

Celsius Temperature: The measurement that can describe extremes of heat. Heat on a scale of 0°C is the stage when water freezes and 100°C is the point water boils at 1 atmosphere (sea level).

Chemical Equation: this refers to the amalgamation or combination of element symbols and formulas to render a chemical reaction of reactants and products.

Chemical Properties: this term refers to a substance's interaction with other substances observed and documented as a substance's behavior under standard conditions.

Coagulation: A condition where a protein in a fluid state becomes insoluble by contact with heat or a chemical as when blood clots within the body. Examples of chemicals that cause this condition are aldehyde or alcohol.

Colloid: A solution which has a charge and consists of tiny particles which are larger than molecular size but small enough to be moved about by molecules. The particles settle through neutralizing the charge, not by gravity.

Combustion: this term refers to the production of heat and light through a process of rapid oxidation as in explosions.

Compound Lipid: A lipid or fat which exists in the blood. The hydrolytic process is the chemical process that occurs when a molecule is cleaved into two parts after being introduced to a molecule of water. Alcohol, fatty acids and other substances when introduced to a molecule of water can begin the hydrolytic process.

Compound: A molecularly and chemically bonded substance which has two or more atoms in proportions to its mass or size.

Compressibility: The volume of a gas decreased by increasing pressure. When the pressure is great enough and the individual molecules of the gas begin to interact with each other, the gas turns to a liquid state.

Concentrated Solution: A substance which contains a high proportion of solute.

Concentration: The ratio of solvent to solute in a solution. The solvent is the medium or chemical used to dissolve a substance and the substance dissolved is the solute.

Condensation: A condition that occurs when a gas turns from the gaseous state into a liquid state usually through a cooling process.

Covalent Bond: The chemical joining that is formed when two atoms share a pair of electrons.

Crystallization: this term refers to the condition that happens when a substance is given a solid form.

Deamination: The condition that occurs when the liver breaks down amino acids. The amino group is removed creating ammonia. The left over in the amino group is the carbon and hydrogen. Carbon and hydrogen are burned by the body for energy. The enzymes within the body add carbon dioxide to the ammonia to make urea or uric acid which is defused into the blood and ultimately excreted by the body.

Decarboxylation: The removal of the COOH carboxyl group from a compound.

Dehydration: The removal of water from matter which can present a dangerous situation to a living being.

Denaturation: Breakdown of a protein's physical properties which cause it to become chemically inactive. This breakdown is accomplished through heat or chemicals.

Density: Ratio of mass to volume or capacity.

Desiccation: this term refers to the loss of water and the drying conditions that result from this process.

Dialdehyde: CHO or the compound which contains two organic aldehyde radicals.

Diffusibility: The movement of gas into the environment it occupies. Gas has no fixed shape or volume.

Diffusion: The action of a substance which seeks to form a uniform or equal concentration in a given area.

Dilute Solution: A solvent with a low ratio of solute.

Disaccharide: Condition that occurs when two single or monosaccharide sugar units link together in order to formulate a carbohydrate sugar.

Emulsion: this term refers to the solution made when two insoluble liquids are mixed together.

Endothermic Reaction: this term refers to a chemical process that absorbs heat from the surroundings or environment.

Energy: this term refers to the capacity of a system to exert itself in work.

Enzyme: this term refers to a protein which causes biological chemical reactions while maintaining its own properties. This ability categorizes it as a catalyst.

Ester: this term refers to the formula RCOOR'. In this formula, R is the symbol that stands for the hydrocarbon group or hydrogen. The R' symbol stands for the hydrocarbon group that is formed from alcohol and an organic or carboxylic acid derived from the removal of water.

Ether: this term refers to the group with an oxygen atom bonded to two alkyl groups. In this group it is the oxygen atom which is responsible for the bonding. The formula: ROR' where R and R' are hydrocarbon groups formed by dehydration process of two alcohols.

Exothermic Reaction: this term refers to the condition that occurs when a substance releases heat into the surrounding area.

Expansivity: The expansion of gas in heat applications. Particles have a minimal interaction with each other as they are far removed from each other with high velocities of movement.

Fat: this term refers to a semisolid or solid triglyceride that is also known as a saturated fatty acid.

Formaldehyde Demand: this term refers to the total amount of HCHO that will coalesce with and completely preserve protein.

Formalin: this term refers to a formaldehyde gas that is dissolved in water.

Formula: this term refers to an expression of symbols which represents a substance's chemical makeup.

Freezing: this term refers to what happens when heat is removed.

Functional Group: this term refers to an atom or group of atoms when attached to a carbon atom in a compound will have a specific chemical performance or function.

Gas: this refers to the state or condition of matter in which the atoms are far apart and have almost complete freedom from one another. Gas assumes the shape of the container in which it is held.

General Formula: this term refers to the symbols which indicate a class of compounds. The compounds with R are indicative of a radical including a functional group.

Glucose: this term refers to a compound which makes up the simple sugar formula: $C_6H_{12}O_6$.

Glycogen: this term refers to an alpha glucose molecule chain which forms an animal starch.

Hard water: this term refers to the condition or state of water which contains minerals and metallic ions.

Hemoglobin: this term refers to the protein in blood that contains iron.

Hexose: this term refers to a 6 carbon sugar molecule such as glucose: $C_6H_{12}O_6$.

Homogeneous: this term refers to a uniform or unwavering composition of matter.

Hydrate: this term refers to a compound formed or produced as water combines with another substance and forms crystals. One example is the infusion of crystallized salts with water.

Hydrocarbon: this term refers to the molecule formed or produced by the combining of hydrogen and carbon together.

Hydrolysis: this term refers to the action of water breaking down a compound as in the action between a salt and water to form an acid and a base composition.

Hypertonic Solution: this term refers to the solution which has a larger concentration.

Hypotonic solution: this term refers to the solution which has a smaller concentration.

Imbibitions: this term refers to the condition that occurs when moisture is infused into the surrounding tissue area. This causes distension and softening of the tissue.

Index: this term refers to the embalming fluid concentration ratio number of formaldehyde gas grams per 100ml of water. For example, the index percentage: 13 indexes is 13% formaldehyde gas.

Ion: this term refers to the negative or positive state of an electrically charged atom or molecule. The positive charge is a cation and the negative charge is an anion.

Ionization: this term is used when molecules are split into cation and anion particles which cause the molecules to either remove the electrons of an atom to become positively charged or it causes the molecules to produce ions in a solution to become negatively charged.

Isomerism: this term is used when two molecules have the exact same number of atoms, but are arranged in a different fashion. However, the chemical properties can be similar or very different from each other.

Isotonic solution: this term refers to the same salt concentration as that of normal human cells and blood. An isotonic cellular environment occurs when there is equal concentration of a solute inside and outside the cell. The cell size stays the same because molecules flow in and out of the cell at an equal rate of speed.

Ketone: this term refers to the matter produced when fat breaks down and accumulates in the blood. This is caused by a lack of sufficient insulin or caloric intake.

Ketose: this term refers to a monosaccharide sugar which has one ketone group with a functional group which is of the hydroxyl OH group. The formula: R1COR2.

Kilogram: this term refers to a metric measurement of 1000 grams.

Kinetic energy: this term refers to the motion of a body which is defined as the work expended to bring a body from the resting state to a motion or active state of being.

Lethal Dose: this is abbreviated as LD and is the quantity of poison or radiation required to kill a proportion equaling one half of the group poisoned.

Lewis base: The compound which tends to donate or give off two electrons.

Line Formula: this term is an abbreviation of formulas written in a symbolic notation which is used to conserve or save space.

Liquefaction: this term refers to a condition that occurs when liquid is formed from a gaseous or a solid substance.

Liquid: this term refers to a material which flows but does not expand to fill its containers space.

Liter: this term refers to a measurement of volume in the metric system for liquids.

Mass: this term is used for the amount of substance. However, this term should not be used in terms of the weight of a substance.

Matter: this term can be used to describe anything that has substance and has the ability to occupy or take up space.

Melting: this term is used when a solid becomes a liquid caused by the dislocation of the crystal lattice which allows the molecules to move about more freely.

Metal: this term is used to refer to a chemical element that is a cation in solution with the appearance that is shiny and pliable. This element can conduct heat and/or electricity.

Metathesis Reaction: this term is used when elements or radicals exchange places in two different compounds due to the driving force which has caused the removal of ions from the solution.

Meter: this term is used in a metric system measurement to describe length.

Minimum Lethal Dose: this term is abbreviated as MLD and is the least amount of a poisonous, deadly measure that has the effect of killing a person.

Mixture: this term is used when two substances are combined without a chemical union of the two.

Molecular Formula: this term refers to the symbols which illustrate the chemical make up of an element that describes the number of atoms in the molecule but doesn't describe how the atoms are bonded or held together.

Molecule: The composition of two or more electrically stable atoms. It is the smallest particle of a substance maintaining the properties of that substance.

Monatomic Ion: this term refers to a single atom which has an electrical charge.

Monosaccharide: this term refers to a sugar in its simplest form and it cannot be decomposed by hydrolysis.

Neutralization: this term refers to the process of making a salt and water from an acid and a base combination.

Neutron: this term refers to the center particle in the atom that has no electrical charge. It has a mass similar to a proton.

Nonmetal: this term refers to any material that will ionize negatively in a solution.

Nucleus: this term refers to the very center of an atom which is positively charged and is densely packed with neutrons and protons.

Oil: this term refers to the triacylglycerol which is a viscous liquid at room temperature with a high concentration of fatty acids.

Osmosis: this refers to when fluid flows from one cell to another in order to dilute the higher concentration to a low concentration of salt. This will flow toward a higher concentration of salt to equalize the concentrations on both sides of the membrane.

Oxidation Number: this refers to the number of electrons that are lost, shared, or gained in a chemical reaction or chemical change.

Oxidation: this refers to the addition of oxygen and removal of hydrogen which stabilizes the substance through the removal of electrons from an element or compound.

Oxide: this term refers to a compound which contains oxygen and one other element.

Pentose: this term refers to a sugar molecule with 5 carbons.

Peptide Bond: this term refers to a link formed between two amino acids during the dehydration process. The amino group of one acid joins with the carboxyl group of the other acid during the dehydration process.

Periodic Table: this term refers to the arrangement of elements according to an atomic numeric increase in such a way as the columns illustrate the elements with similar properties.

Permanent Hardness of Water: this occurs when carbonates from calcium and magnesium (chloride and sulfate) are in the water. The only way to remove this condition is by adding other chemicals.

pH: this refers to the measurement of hydrogen ions in a solution on a scale from 0 to 14. The measurement of 7 is neutral and when measurement is below 7 there is a more acidic count. A measurement above 7 is considered a basic measurement.

Physical Change: this occurs when there is a form transformation with a change in chemical composition.

Poison: this term refers to a substance which is toxic to the body and has the potential to endanger a person's life or health.

Polyatomic Ion: this term refers to a complex of atoms which have an electrical charge. These atoms act as a molecule or as a single unit. Radicals are free agents which do not have an electrical charge along with an unpaired electron.

Polymer: this term refers to a substance formed by bonding several monomers or basic chemical units through a process called polymerization.

Polysaccharide: this term refers to a polymer of simple sugar molecules. Examples of these are starch or cellulose.

Potential energy: this term refers to stored up energy matter.

Precipitate: this term refers to the matter in a solution which is insoluble or only partially soluble.

Pre-injection Fluid: this term refers to the blood's cleansing solution that flows through the vascular system and makes the arterial solution distributed with greater efficiency.

Preservatives: this refers to the embalming fluids which are the reactants that interfere with decomposition. This interference can stop the chemical reactions between amino acids and proteins, kill microorganisms, remove odors, eliminate enzyme formations, and deactivate the enzymes present.

Pressure: this refers to the force exerted upon the surface of a unit area or region.

Primary Alcohol: this term refers to the OH group attached to a carbon.

Protein: this term refers to the substance composed of amino acids.

Proton: this term refers to the positively charged particle in the atom with a mass number of 1 and the electrical charge is +1.

Putrefaction: this term refers to the decomposition of organic material in which amines have produced an offensive stench which is typically caused by putrescine and/or cadaverine.

Quaternary Ammonium Compound: this term refers to a disinfectant used on the surface of skin, nasal and oral cavities or on outer work surfaces. An example of one such surface would be the tools which are disinfected with a germicide solution.

Reduction: this term refers to the decrease of oxidation number used to track electrons during a redox reaction. An increase in the number means that electrons have been lost and oxidation has occurred. A decrease indicates a reduction and those electrons have been gained.

Restorative Fluids: this term refers to liquids used to remove discolorations or those which reduce moisture in the tissues or replace moisture in the tissues for cosmetic reasons or purposes.

Salt: this term refers to the substance produced when acids and bases chemically react.

Saturated Hydrocarbon: this refers to the single bonded hydrocarbons.

Saturated Solution: this term refers to the solvent which is unable to dissolve any more solute than it already has done so at a particular temperature and pressure.

Secondary Alcohol: this term refers to a hydroxyl group in which the OH group is linked to a carbon linked to two other carbons.

Simple Lipid: this term refers to a water molecule which is added to another molecule which causes a division of that other molecule to create fatty acids and alcohols.

Single Replacement Reaction: this occurs when a free element is substituted for one of the elements in a compound. For example: a solution of an ionic compound has an available element that replaces one of the ions; this introduces a new element from the ion solution.

Solid: this term refers to the matter in a state of denseness which has neither a gaseous or fluid construction.

Solidification: this term refers to the process of making a substance hard or dense in form.

Solubility: this term refers to the ability of a substance to dissolve in another substance.

Solute: this term refers to the substance dissolved in a solvent to form or make a solution in which the solute is in a lesser amount than the solvent.

Specific gravity: this term refers to the ratio of density which uses water as the standard to measure the ratio.

Stereoisomerism: this term refers to the bonding process that is the same but allows for the geometrical position of atoms and functional groups to be different. When two stereoisomers are mirror images of each other, then they are enantiomers with identical chemical and physical properties. They are symmetrical and rotate in opposite directions from each other. The enzymes can differentiate between the two stereoisomers and will often prefer one stereoisomer over another.

Structural Formula: this term refers to a display of atoms where each atomic link and arrangement in their chemical make up is a depiction of that bond or link.

Structural Isomerism: this term refers to the functional groups that are joined in the hydrocarbon chains with different branching in dissimilar fashions.

Sublimation: Refers to when matter changes from the solid state directly into the gaseous state. One inhibitor of this process is caused by the heating of iodine crystals. When the heat is applied, the crystals change into purple gas and when the heat is removed, the gas forms back into crystals.

Substrate: this term refers to a molecule that an enzyme catalyzes as a result of a chemical reaction.

Supplementary Germicide: this term refers to the additive in the embalming fluid which is designed to kill infectious microorganisms.

Surface Tension: this term refers to the attraction or pull of molecules to each other that make a barrier or molecular film between air and the underlying molecules of the liquid.

Surfactant: this term refers to any substance which reduces or lessens the surface tension in such a way that the membranes cause a barrier to diffuse the embalming fluids in the tissues.

Suspension: this occurs when particles of the solute are greater than 100 nanometers in size. These particles are large enough to keep from passing through a filter or membrane, but small enough to mix in the solvent without settling.

Symbol: this term refers to the chemical element abbreviation that represents the chemical element.

Temporary Hardness of Water: Occurs when boiling produces a decomposition reaction which converts or changes the bicarbonate salts of calcium and magnesium into insoluble substances.

Tertiary Alcohol: this occurs when the OH group is attached to a carbon attached to three other carbons.

Thioalcohol: this term is also known as Mercaptan which is a compound where oxygen in a hydroxyl group OH, is replaced by a sulfur atom SHH

Toxin: this term refers to a poisonous substance produced by a plant, animal, or bacteria which is categorized as a protein or conjugated protein.

Triacylglycerol: this term refers to a lipid water molecule which cleaves to and divides another molecule with three fatty acids and glycerol which are typically known as triglycerides or neutral fats.

True Solution: this term refers to a molecular mixture of a homogenous nature where the particles are of 1 nanometer in size allowing the substances to pass through membranes.

Unsaturated Solution: this term refers to a solvent which can absorb and dissolve more solute into itself under a particular or given temperature and pressure.

Vapor: this term refers to a gaseous state of a substance which given normal or ordinary temperatures, the substance would be in the form of a solid or liquid.

Vaporization: this term refers to the process of converting a liquid to a gaseous state or form.

Viscosity: this term refers to the measure of a liquid's internal friction or its ability to flow or be able to resist the flow. In most circumstances, the higher the temperature, the lower the viscosity. For example: heated molasses flows quicker than cold molasses. Cold molasses has a high viscosity rate.

Volatile: this term refers to a chemical ability to convert from liquid to gaseous state or forms.

Wax: this term refers to a compound composed or made from unsaturated and/or saturated fatty acids and alcohols which are not glycerin.

Weight: this term refers to a measurement of gravitational pull on a mass which makes it dependent upon its position in a gravitational field.

Anatomy and Physiology

Anatomy is a term which comes from the Greek words *anatomia* and *anatemnein* which means to cut up or to cut open. Anatomy has three major subsections: comparative anatomy, histology, human anatomy. The embalmer is concerned with the human body's system and the structures of the vascular system, organs, muscular, skeletal, and lymphatic and nervous systems. The embalmer concentrates on the vascular system which disburses the embalming fluids throughout the body.

Physiology includes the study of the endocrine system, its interaction with the nervous system, and the secretions or hormones that regulate the body's systems. Organs, tissues and cells interact with each other on a chemical level as well as a physical level. Physiology focuses on function and the effects of nutrition, metabolism, and transport. The embalmer uses his or her understanding of physiology in using embalming fluids which cause chemical reactions in the body.

The Blood

Blood has a specific chemical composition. The pH level of blood is slightly alkaline, 7.34 to 7.45, which allow the body's enzymes to function at optimum levels. If the blood becomes too acidic, the condition can cause the death of the person. Blood has a viscosity of approximately 3.3 to 5.5 which is three to five times thicker than water. Blood is a circulating tissue composed of plasma and cells. Because of its origin in the bones and its function, blood is known as a connective tissue. The main function of blood is to supply nutrients throughout the body. In addition, blood carries waste to purification centers to be excreted out of the body. Blood transports cells and other substances between tissues and organs. Any abnormalities or anomalies found in the blood will lead to tissue dysfunction. Tissue dysfunction can lead to illness or death.

Other terms

Albumins: this term refers to the protein types which are manufactured in the liver. These are responsible for transporting water in the blood which preserves blood volume. These proteins make up about 60% of the plasma. When the number of albumins decreases, edema occurs in tissues.

Fibrinogen: this term refers to the protein which helps the blood to clot in the body.

Globulins: this term refers to alpha and beta globulins which convey fats in the bloodstream. LDL or low density lipoproteins carry cholesterol from the liver to the body cells, and HDL or high density lipoproteins remove cholesterol from the arteries. Gamma globulins act as antibodies in five categories: IgA, IgD, IgE, IgG, and IgM which have explicit method of immune system defense.

Plasma: the main function is to exchange dissolved substances through the endothelium lining of the blood vessels to the tissue underneath. Nutrients are deposited and waste is extracted. Wastes consists of 90% water, 7% blood proteins, and 3% is composed of hormones, electrolytes, amino acids, enzymes, nutrients and other waste products. Plasma proteins are albumins, globulins and fibrinogens.

Serotonin: this term refers is a chemical found in the thrombocytes platelets. This chemical is a vasoconstrictor and its reaction helps to stem blood loss within the body.

Thrombocytes: this term refers to the platelets which are flat and disc-shaped filled with enzymes. These platelets help in blood clotting and plugging in the damaged places in blood vessels by clustering together to form a patch, or barrier. This barrier allows the blood vessel to heal. These platelets contain proteins, actin and myosin, which reduce the mass of the clot. This promotes healing by also pulling the edges of the hole together to decrease blood loss.

The Heart

The heart is located in the middle of the chest behind the sternum (mediastinum) and is located slightly to the left of that area. The three layers of the heart wall are the epicardium, myocardium and the endocardium. The outer layer is the visceral pericardium or epicardium. The outer layer is covered with fat, adipose tissue, and contains coronary blood vessels. These vessels act as conduits that drain blood away from the heart. Cardiac muscle is in the myocardium, the middle layer of the heart, along with connective tissue, blood vessels and nerves. The endocardium is the innermost layer and is similar to the endothelium of blood vessels. Research shows that this inner most layer actually control the myocardial function. This is particularly true when the heart is in the embryo state. The innermost layer controls the development of the heart within the body.

Coronary arteries are tubes which supply blood to the myocardium: veins drain the blood; left and right branches of the ascending aorta are the coronary arteries which bring blood to the myocardium; then the blood flows from the myocardium in the middle and great cardiac veins, and flows into the cardiac capillaries to the coronary sinus vein. **The cardiac septum** is a wall that separates the left side of the heart from the right; *interatrial septum* divides left and right atriums; *interventricular septum* divides left and right ventricles. The **right atrium** is a portion of the heart, plays a crucial role in drainage during embalming: blood leaves the right atrium and enters the right ventricle. **The right ventricle** is the point where blood enters and goes through the *right atrioventricular orifice* (holds the *right atrioventricular valve,* which prevents back flow into the right atrium); blood is pumped from the right ventricle through the pulmonary trunk orifice that leads to the pulmonary arteries; to prevent back flow, the pulmonary semilunar valve closes. The **interatrial septum** is a wall of the right atrium section where the fossa ovalis lies. This is a leftover from fetal circulation (foramen ovale). The fetus receives oxygenated blood from the umbilical cord from the mother so the right ventricle is bypassed through the hole in interatrial septum. The foramen ovale closes over after birth because of the left atrium pressure and this becomes the fossa ovalis in the adult.

Major arteries

Starting at the head of the right side of the body the major arteries include: the anterior cerebral, middle cerebral, basilar, internal carotid, external carotid, vertebral, right common carotid, right subclavian, axillary, innominate (brachiocephalic), brachial, radial, interosseous, ulnar, deep palmar arch, superficial palmar arch, digital arteries, left subclavian, celiac, splenic, superior mesenteric, renal, aorta, inferior mesenteric, external iliac, internal iliac, common femoral, deep femoral, superficial femoral, popliteal, peroneal, anterior tibial, posterior tibial, and ends at the toes on the left side of the body with the dorsalis pedis.

Starting at the head of the right side of the body the major veins include: Head: Superior sagittal sinus, straight sinus, external jugular, internal jugular, right innominate, Deep Arm veins: subclavian, axillary, profunda brachial, brachial, radial, interosseous, ulnar; Superficial arm veins: Cephalic, basilica, median cubital, digital; Torso: Left innominate, superior vena cava, hepatic, renal, inferior vena cava, common iliac, internal iliac; Leg veins: external iliac, common femoral, profunda femoris, superficial femoral, popliteal, anterior tibial, peroneal, posterior tibial; superficial leg veins: greater saphenous, and ends at the lesser saphenous.

Other terms

Left Ventricle: The most powerful chamber in the heart. The left atrioventricular is often called the mitral valve and the bicuspid valve because it has two cusps instead of three. The blood then leaves the left ventricle and passes through the aortic orifice into the ascending aorta and the aortic semilunar valve stops any back flow.

Lumen: The open space in which blood flows in the vessel.

Pericardial Sac: this is the section that surrounds the heart in three distinct parts: visceral pericardium (epicardium) and the parietal pericardium. The visceral pericardium covers the surface of the heart. The parietal pericardium is the lining of the pericardial sac. The fibrous pericardium has collagen fibers and is the outer most membrane of the sac. The functions of this sac promotes cardiac efficiency by distributing hydrostatic forces and creates a closed chamber which promotes healthy cardiac pressure and shields it from external friction and infection.

Pulmonary Veins: The four veins or tubes which deposit the blood into the left atrium. Blood goes through the pulmonary venous orifices and the left atrioventricular orifice to the atrioventricular valve and the blood then passes through to the left ventricle.

Tunica Externa: The outer layer or tunica adventitia which forms the connective tissue sheath around the vessels. This sheath bonds with the surrounding tissue locking the vessels in place.

Tunica Interna: The innermost layer of the endothelial lining. It has an elastic fibrous connective tissue. Arteries have an elastic membrane that veins do not have.

Tunica Media: The middle layer of muscles within connective tissue. This layer secures the blood vessels together. This layer is responsible for the constriction of the muscles. When constricted the size of the lumen is slowed. When the muscles relax, the lumen widens and blood flow increases and speeds up.

The Digestive System

The biochemical properties of the digestive system affect the embalming process and affect the decomposition process. The digestive system is made up of the alimentary canal which is the mouth, pharynx, esophagus, stomach, small intestine, large intestine, rectum and anus. The mouth is the first digestive process when food or drink is mixed with saliva by the grinding action of the teeth. The mouth has hard and soft palates on the roof. The hard palate is the maxillary bone and the palate bones. Dangling tissues found at the back of the mouth form the uvula which prevents food from going down the pharynx before it should. The pharynx has three sections: nasopharynx, oropharynx and laryngopharynx. The nasopharynx is above the soft palate. The oropharynx is between the soft palate and the epiglottis. The laryngopharynx is behind the epiglottis which is linked to the esophagus or the throat.

Esophagus to the stomach

The digestive system's esophagus uses mucus to lubricate. The bolus or chewed up food slides down the esophagus with ease. The sphincter muscles are found at the top and bottom of the esophagus. They close off during peristalsis, wave-like muscular motion that pushes the food through the digestive tract. Below the diaphragm, the digestive system is known as the gastrointestinal tract, or GI. The parts of the digestive tract begin at the salivary glands, oral cavity, teeth, tongue, pharynx, esophagus, liver, stomach, gallbladder, pancreas, large intestine, small intestine, appendix, rectum. The stomach or the gaster is a sac that is protected by the left rib cage and below the diaphragm. It produces hydrochloric acid to digest food for the next organ along the digestive tract. The ridges of muscles go along in three directions of fibers which are longitudinal, circular and oblique.

Rugae to the ileum

The stomach has many folds in the mucous membrane lining or the rugae. As the stomach churns the food with the gastric juices it creates a liquid called chyme. Digestive enzymes are lipase and pepsinogen. The chyme travels to the small intestine. The small intestine has three sections: duodenum, the jejunum, and the ileum. The duodenum is a jointed tube that links the stomach to the jejunum. The jejunum then secretes mucous and breaks down the chyme. The jejunum is several feet long and the lining is covered in villi which help absorb nutrients inside the intestine. The ileum is separated from the cecum of the large intestine by the ileocecal valve. The ileum has a huge amount of microvilli on the epithelial cells which absorb vitamin B_{12} and bile salts.

Large intestine to descending colon

The next stage of the digestive system is found in the large intestine. The large intestine absorbs water and packs the undigested chyme into feces. The large intestines have three sections: cecum, colon and rectum. Cecum is a sac with a tail called the appendix which contains lymphoid tissue that helps the immune response. The cecum contains huge numbers of microorganisms and must be cleaned thoroughly by the embalmer because these microorganisms will speed up the decomposition of the remains. The colon has 4 sections: ascending, transverse, descending and the sigmoid. The ascending section extends up to the liver and makes a 90° turn called the hepatic flexure. The transverse crosses over the abdomen to the spleen then becomes a downward turn called the left splenic flexure. The descending colon goes down to the rim of the pelvis.

Descending colon to rectum

The next stage of the digestive system begins at the descending colon and takes an S-shaped turn into the sigmoid colon. Then it goes across the pelvis to the middle of the sacrum and links to the rectum. The rectum follows along the vertebra sacrum and coccyx to the anal canal. The anus contains the internal sphincter and external anal sphincter. The interior sphincter remains closed and the external is a voluntary-controlled muscle. When muscles relax after death, these muscles may allow intestinal purge to leak. Packing the anus with cavity-soaked cotton is a standard practice of the embalmer.

Other terms

Gallbladder: this term refers to the cholecyst which is pear-shaped and is found next to the visceral wall of the liver. This organ stores bile produced by the liver. The small intestine secretes a hormone called cholecystokinin which opens the sphincter and the gallbladder contracts causing bile to flow through the ducts into the duodenum of the large intestine.

Mastication: this term refers to the act of chewing food.

Pancreas: this term refers to the organ which is heterocrine. Heterocrine indicates the two kinds of glandular tissue found in the pancreas: endocrine and exocrine. The endocrine releases insulin which metabolizes sugar. Pancreatic juice is secreted which contains water, ions, digestive enzymes and buffers that control the pH levels. This juice breaks down the chyme or chunks of food through hydrolysis.

Salivary glands: this term refers to the three glands which begin the chemical process for breaking down food. The three glands include: sublingual salivary glands, the parotid salivary glands and the submandibular salivary glands. The submandibular salivary glands are located under the tongue, near the ear and along the mandible.

Teeth: 32 teeth in the adult human which can tear and grind food into swallow-able sized pieces.

Tongue: this term refers to a muscle covered in papillae. The connective tissue under the tongue is the lingual frenum and at the base are Warton's ducts. These ducts release saliva. Liver: this term refers to the organ responsible for metabolic functions, hematological functions, storage functions and bile-related functions. The lobule is a central vein that works as the center unit within the liver. Kupffer cells filter the blood and destroy worn out red blood cells, white blood cells and microorganisms and toxins. It regulates blood sugar. It will store glucose in the form of glycogen when there is too much blood sugar. The glycogenolysis process occurs as glucose is converted to raise the blood sugar levels. This system manufactures lipoproteins, cholesterol and phospholipids by using fats. It formulates ketone bodies. Plasma proteins and albumins are synthesized. This allows the removal of pathogens and damaged cells. Bile salts are manufactured and secreted into the duodenum. The detoxification of the body is easily affected by pathological conditions.

The Respiratory System

Respiratory system refers to the system or coordinated effort that brings oxygen into and throughout the body. The process of inhaling and exhaling air is known as ventilation. When oxygen is exchanged for the carbon dioxide waste, it is called respiration which is external in the lungs and accomplished internally in the blood. The body performs this in a relatively involuntary manner. The body can sustain life without water and food for long periods, but oxygen is vital. Oxygen can be cut off for only a few minutes without causing damage or death to the person.

The lungs

The lungs are the part of the respiratory system that has a network of bronchioles and alveoli. Oxygen diffuses from the air through alveoli membrane into the blood and the carbon dioxide diffuses from the blood into the alveoli, to the air, and out of the system in this exchange. The left and right lungs serve as a spongy cushion for the heart as they are formed around the heart organ. The left lung is longer and narrower and has only two lobes. The heart is right in the location that a third lobe would be if it existed. The right lung has three lobes. Each lung has a hilus on the medial surface used for the entry and exit point for the bronchiole tubes, pulmonary blood vessels, lymphatic vessels and nerves. The visceral pleura slides along the parietal pleura separated by a pleural space filled with fluid.

Other terms

Alveoli: this is part of the respiratory system where the gaseous oxygen and carbon dioxide exchange takes place. These microscopic sacs provide surface area that is 20 times larger than skin. The capillaries which surround each alveolus are so small that blood cells pass one at a time.

Bronchi: this is part of the respiratory system that is divided by the trachea into left and right bronchi. In the right, there are three bronchioles branches and in the left are two. In each bronchiole there are numerous branches which divide off into smaller and smaller bronchioles. These smaller bronchioles lead to the alveolar ducts connected to alveoli or the microscopic sacs.

Trachea: this is part of the respiratory system which is made of sixteen to twenty cartilaginous rings and is anterior to the esophagus. Longitudinal muscle and elastic cartilage run the length of the trachea so that it easily bends and stretches. The C-shaped rings are open toward the back of the trachea which allows for the esophagus to extend during peristalsis. Ciliated epithelial cells line the trachea, which push mucus laden with foreign particles to the pharynx. Particles such as dust and microbes found are then swallowed or spit out.

The Urinary System

The urinary system functions to remove toxins from the body in a fluid state or form. The urinary system is responsible to maintain and to keeps the body fluids at optimum levels within the body. This balance is regulated by a delicate system. Blood volume is regulated by the balance of the water level in the human body. The blood volumes are responsible for regulating the blood pressure of the body. For this reason, the urinary system also eliminates any drug and/or alcohol toxins from the body. The urinary system plays a crucial role in maintenance of the pH balances within the tissues. The organs which make up the urinary system include: the kidneys, ureters, bladder and urethra. Two tubes called ureters descend from the kidneys to the bladder. The bladder is the sac that holds urine for voluntary excretion. The urethra empties the bladder to the outside of the body.

Blood is filtered. The plasma filtered out by the glomerulus is glomerular filtrate. Glomerular filtrate is the combination of water that has electrolytes, sugars, urea, amino acids, polypeptides and other solutes. The proximal convoluted tubule is lined with cuboidal epithelial cells which have microvilli. It is the microvilli that absorb some water, electrolytes, sugar and select amino acids and polypeptides, the rest is passed through the Loop of Henle. This solution becomes either more or less concentrated depending upon the amount of the hormone released by the anterior pituitary gland. The pituitary gland lets the body know if there is a need for more or less water. The urine then travels into the medulla through a collecting duct into a minor calyx. It then travels from there to one of the major calyces that discards or empties it into the renal pelvis.

Other terms

Bladder: this term refers to the sac that holds urine for voluntary excretion. It is muscular and has three layers: tunica mucosa, tunica muscularis, and tunica serosa. The tunica mucosa is the epithelium that folds when the bladder is empty of urine. The tunica muscularis has three tracks of muscle fibrous material. The tunica serosa is the outer layer or coating which works to secrete friction reducing lubricants.

Bulbourethral Gland: this term refers to the gland which prevents urine from entering the penis during sexual intercourse.

Glomerular Capsule: this term refers to the connection to the medulla by a tubule which is known as the Loop of Henle. This tube loops back toward the cortex as the distal convoluted tubule that is found near the proximal convoluted tubule. Then it joins with the collecting tubules that empty distilled urine into the renal pelvis.

Glomerulus: this term refers to a capillary clump that receives blood from an arteriole that carries blood back to the center of renal circulation. The blood pressure in the glomerulus is what forces the filtration of fluid and removal of the undesirable solutes produced by metabolism. The nitrogenous wastes of urea and uric acid are removed.

Nephron: this term refers to the most basic unit found within the kidney. These units number in the millions and are found in each kidney. These units function to filter and regulate the water level in the body tissues. Nephrons give off signals to begin the reabsorption or excretion of water processes.

Perirenal Fat: this term refers to the renal capsule found in the kidneys.

Renal Artery: this term refers to the branch of the abdominal aorta that supplies blood to the kidneys. The vena cava receives blood from the renal vein which drains blood from the kidneys. About 1/1000th of blood filtered through the kidneys is turned into urine, but ¼ of all blood pumped by the heart each minute is filtrated by the kidneys.

Renal Corpuscle: this term refers to the beginning filter of the nephron.

Renal Cortex: this term refers to one of the three parts of the kidneys. This part is the outer layer which is located over the medulla containing the urinary tubes, glomeruli or filters, and blood vessels, all supported by a fibrous tissue within the kidney.

Renal Fascia: this term refers to the fibrous connective tissue which covers or surrounds the kidney organs.

Renal Glands: this term is also known as the kidneys. The kidneys are bean-shaped and are located just above the waistband in the back, one on each side of the spinal column between vertebrae T12 and L3. The right kidney is situated next to the liver and is slightly lower than the left kidney. Both are located behind the stomach, spleen and pancreas.

Renal Pelvis: this term refers to one of the three parts of the kidneys. This part contains the major and minor calyces. It is here that urine is collected before it trickles into the ureters. The ureters are found in the center of the kidney.

The Nervous System

Divisions

The two divisions of the nervous system are the Central Nervous System and the Peripheral Nervous System. CNS is an abbreviation of the term Central Nervous System. CNS is made up of the brain and the spinal cord which functions to receive and send signals throughout the body. PNS is an abbreviation of the term Peripheral Nervous System. PNS is the sensory and motor nervous systems of the body. This system consists of cranial and spinal nerves which work as the transmitters of nervous impulses to the brain and spinal cord. The sensory nervous system is also known as the afferent nervous system because it carries information from the organs back to the central nervous system. The motor nervous system is also known as the efferent nervous system because it carries messages from the brain and spinal cord to the muscles and organs of the body.

Spinal cord

The spinal cord is part of the central nervous system or CNS. The spinal cord runs through the magnum foramen to the first lumbar vertebrae then the roots branch forming the cauda equina. The cord is encased in the protective substance of cerebrospinal fluid. Nerve fibers called funiculi make up the three columns that are positioned along the length of the cord. The columns are named Ventral/Anterior Column, Dorsal/Posterior Column and Lateral Column. This white matter found in the spinal cord is called funiculus. The descending tracts are the motor fibers. The ascending tracts are the sensory fibers. Spinal nerves in the peripheral nervous system are located throughout the entire body's system. The body has 12 cranial nerves in the PNS which are attached to the brain stem. These cranial nerves are also located throughout the body with the exception of the olfactory nerves and optic nerve.

12 Cranial Nerves

The 12 Cranial Nerves are the olfactory nerve, the optic nerve, the oculomotor nerve, the trochlear nerve, the trigeminal nerve, the abducens nerve, the facial nerve, the vestibulocochlear nerve, glossopharyngeal nerve, the vagus nerve, the accessory nerve, and the hypoglossal nerve. Olfactory nerve: this nerve is responsible for the sense of smell. Optic nerve: this nerve is responsible for vision. Oculomotor nerve: this nerve is responsible for the lens and pupil motor control of the eyes. Trochlear nerve: this nerve is responsible for the inferior and lateral eye muscle control movements. Trigeminal: this nerve commands chewing, lip, cheek and eyeball sensations or feelings. Abducens nerve: this nerve is responsible for the lateral motor control of eyeball muscles in the eye. Facial nerve: this nerve is responsible for taste and facial muscles in the face. Vestibulocochlear nerve: this nerve is responsible for hearing and balance. Glossopharyngeal nerve: this nerve is responsible for tongue sensations and controls swallowing. Vagus nerve: this term is responsible for the respiratory system and digestive system sensations. Accessory nerve: this term is responsible for the head/neck movement and voice production. Hypoglossal nerve: this term is responsible for the tongue movement in speech and swallowing.

Other terms

Axon: this term refers to a cable-like projection from the soma which extends less than 1mm or from the spinal cord to the foot. This carries nerve signals and it usually has many branches to communicate with numerous cells.

Brain Divisions: this term refers to the three divisions of the brain. These divisions are the cerebrum, the cerebellum and the brain stem.

Brain Stem: this term refers to the part of the brain which sends the messages and contains the midbrain, pons, and medulla oblongata. These allow muscle movement and perception of sensory input.

Cerebellum: this term refers to the section of the brain which is in charge of bodily motor functions and sensations. This part of the brain works to harmonize muscle movements and monitors position of body parts for optimal performance.

Cerebrum: this term refers to the section of the brain which is covered by a thin outer layer called the cerebral cortex. Hills in this section are called gyri. The valleys are called sulci. Each side of the cerebrum controls the opposite side of the body. They link together at the clump of axons called the corpus callosum. The five lobes of the cerebrum are frontal, parietal, temporal, occipital, and insula. The frontal section is responsible for speech and moral values. The parietal is responsible for the five senses input. The temporal is responsible for the hearing, balance, and emotional responses. The occipital is responsible for vision. The insula is responsible for gastrointestinal and visceral responses.

Dendrite: this term refers to branching cellular extensions similar to tree branches called the dendritic tree. This tree is considered the major reception network of the cell.

Hypothalamus: this term refers to the portion of the brain which normalizes homeostasis. Homeostasis is the body's ability to keep physiological and psychological stability. The hypothalamus regulates temperature, metabolism, blood sugar levels, and senses hunger, thirst, and feelings of satiation or fullness.

Meninges: this term refers to the three protective membranes that cover the brain and spinal cord. The first membrane or the outermost is called the dura mater. Dura mater has two layers of tissue lining the inside of the skull and the vertebral foramen. The second is called the arachnoid membrane and is the center membrane that covers the brain and spinal cord like a spider's web. The third is called the pia mater and is thin and covers the surface of the brain and the spinal cord. The pia mater holds most of the blood vessels which carry blood and oxygen to the brain.

Myelin: this term refers to the fatty, phospholipid matter that covers the axon of some neurons in a cell.

Neurofilaments: this term refers to the structure found in the mitochondria of the cell.

Neurons: this term refers to the nerve cells and is the basic functional unit of the nervous tissue. Nerves are clumps of neurons massed together and are comprised of three parts: soma, axon and dendrites.

Neurotransmitters: this term refers to the transmitter which is found in the space between neurons. This space is called a neuromuscular junction and a neurotransmitter is the chemical that links at the receptor site. It is at this site that the chemical is released from the bulb at the end of the axon. One example of a common transmitter is acetylcholine.

Neurotubules: this term refers to the transmitting proteins found in the mitochondria of the cell.

Soma: this term refers to the cell body which consists of the nucleus, endoplasmic reticulum, lysosomes, mitochondria, neurotubules, and neurofilaments.

Thalamus: this term refers to the portion of the brain located in the cerebrum's diencephalon or the posterior portion of the forebrain and connects the cerebral hemispheres with the mesencephalon. This portion deciphers the senses and controls voluntary muscle movement according to the code given it from the senses.

Ventricles: this term refers to the four cavities in the brain and one in the brain stem that contain cerebrospinal fluid.

Reproduction

Female reproductive system terms

Ovaries: this term refers to the stroma or the inner layer of the female reproductive system which has follicles that hold the eggs or oocytes. The follicles are called graafian follicles. When the egg is mature, it is released into the outer layer or germinal layer. The corpus luteum is tissue which releases the hormones that determines when the eggs are released.

Fallopian Tubes: this term refers to the connection between the ovary and the uterus which allows the egg to travel to the uterus.

Fetus: the unborn baby inside the placenta held in the uterus.

Mammary Glands: this term refers to the ducts which secrete milk for the nourishment of the baby.

Sex Hormones: this term refers to estrogen and progesterone which cause female sex traits to develop and regulates the menses of the female. The hormone, human chorionic gonadotropin, keeps the uterus lining intact when an egg is fertilized.

Uterus: this term refers to the organ which houses the developing fetus. When the egg is not fertilized, the stratum functionalis layer of the endometrium is sloughed off each month in the menstrual cycle. This cycle also carries away the blood and glandular secretions through the cervix and vagina.

Vagina: this term refers to the interior of the cervix and posterior to the bladder. This is the birth canal during childbirth. This is also the depository for sperm during intercourse. The final use is as a funnel for menstrual tissue excretions.

Male reproductive system terms

Epididymis: this term refers to the organ which stores sperm and provides the duct system from the testes to the vas deferens to the ejaculatory duct.

Penis: this term refers to the organ which removes urine and ejaculates sperm. The CNS or central nervous system is responsible for controlling erections of the penis. The hypothalamus and sacral plexus of the spinal cord cause parasympathetic vasodilatation of the arterioles and blood flows into the arteries of the penis which flows into the erectile tissues and the engorged tissues compress the veins of the penis causing an erection.

Spermatic Cord: this term refers to the area which stores the sperm prior to ejaculation.

Testicles: this term refers to the organ which produces the sperm in males. Each testicle has an outer fibrous sac called tunica albuginea. This same type of sac can be found surrounding each ovary in the female. The testicle has about 800 seminiferous tubules that produce sperm and help the sperm to mature. Androgens or sex hormones are produced in the testicles.

The Skeletal System

Associated histology

Bone is dense and osseous tissue which is comprised of inorganic salts. Examples of inorganic salts are calcium phosphate and calcium carbonate. These salts give bones their hard structure. The osseous tissue is surrounded by a fibrous matrix. It has a leather-like consistency when the inorganic salts are removed. Aged bones are more brittle. For this reason, aged persons can suffer from fractures as the bone grows more brittle. The elderly are very susceptible to broken bones. In normal functioning, bones produce blood and store these inorganic salts for the body's use. The bone supports the body and protects the visceral organs. The bone works to help provide leverage to the muscles and the tendons.

The skull

The skull is comprised of 29 bones found in the neurocranium, the splanchnocranium, and the temporal bones. Neurocranium has eight bones. Splanchnocranium has 14 bones. There are six temporal bones which contain the ear ossicles. The anatomical position of the skull is the Frankfurt Plane. The Frankfurt Plane is also called the auricula-orbital plane which is the plane which passes through the left orbit and the upper margin of each ear canal. Another name for the ear canal is the porion. It is the canal that is most in parallel to the earth's surface. The skull bones are the frontal, the parietal, the temporal, the occipital, the sphenoid, the ethmoid, the zygomatic, the maxilla, the nasal, the mandible, the palatine, the lacrimal, the vomer, the inferior and the nasal conchae. The bones located in the middle ear are called: malleus, incus, stapes or the hammer, anvil and stirrup.

Other terms

Ankle: the bones found in the ankle are calcaneus, talus, navicular, medial cuneiform, intermediate cuneiform, lateral cuneiform, and cuboidal.

Digits: this refers to the three bones known as the distal, the middle, and the proximal bones which are found in the fingers. Two are found in the thumb.

Femur: this term refers to the thighbone attached to the pelvis found in the leg.

Fibula: this term refers to the calf bone found in the leg.

Hallux: this term refers to the big toe bones found in the foot.

Humerus: this refers to the bone found in the upper arm.

Ilium: this term refers to the upper broad winged bones found in the pelvic girdle.

Ischium: this term refers to the bone which is found in the pelvic girdle at the lower part of the loops.

Metacarpus: this term refers to the 5 bones which are located in the palm of the hand.

Metatarsus: this term refers to the five long bones found in the foot.

Patella: this term refers to the knee cap in the leg.

Pelvic Girdle: this term refers to the three bones known as the ilium, the pubis, and the ischium.

Phalanges: this term refers to the proximal, intermediate and distal bones found in the foot. The hallux has two phalanges and each of the other four toes has three phalanges. The phalanges have sesamoid bones which are ossified nodes in tendons that help with leverage and pressure reduction.

Phalanx: this term refers to the 14 bones found in the hand.

Pubis: this term refers to bone in the middle and at the top part of the lower loops found in the pelvic girdle.

Radius: this term refers to an additional bone found in the lower arm.

Sesamoid: this term refers to the bones that are small ossified nodes found in the tendons which help with leverage and reduce the pressure.

Shoulder girdle: this term refers to the clavicle and scapula bones found in the upper portion of the body or the shoulder area.

Thorax: this term refers to the 24 pairs of ribs attached to the vertebral column. The first 7 pairs are connected to the sternum. The eighth, ninth and tenth are connected by cartilage to the anterior. The eleventh and twelfth are also known as "floating ribs". This name has been given to them because they are not attached in the front.

Tibia: this term refers to the shin bone found in the leg.

Ulna: this term refers to the bone found in the lower arm.

Vertebra: this term refers to the four regions known as the following: cervical (C1-C7), thoracic (T1-T12), lumbar (L1-L5) and sacral—fused (S1-S5), coccygeal (Co1-Co5). The numbers are used to indicate where the bones are located.

Wrist: the bones found in the wrist are the scaphoid, the lunate, the triquetrum, the pisiform, the trapezium, the trapezoid, the capitate, and the hamate.

Lymphatic System

The lymphatic system refers to the vessels that move fluid in one direction from tissues to the blood system. The thoracic duct conducts lymph from the body below the diaphragm and from the left side above the diaphragm. It begins in the cisterna chili and it is added back to the blood stream through the left subclavian vein near the left internal jugular.

Other terms

Adrenal Glands: this organ is located in the superior aspect of the kidneys and they release adrenaline. The adrenalines released are epinephrine and norepinephrine. These adrenalines increase heart rate and blood pressure in the body.

Gut-associate Lymphoid Tissues: this term is abbreviated as GALT and refers to tissues found in the ileum of the small intestine.

Lymph Nodes: this term refers to the lymphoid organs found all over the body.

Lymphoid Tissues: this term refers to the lymphocytes which are embedded in epithelial tissues in the respiratory, digestive and urinary tracts.

Necrobiosis: this term refers to the process where the old cells die and drop off to be replaced by cells from the lower layers. Stratum lucidum and stratum granulosum have proteins which promote hair and nail growth.

Parathyroid Glands: this organ is located in the thyroid gland lobes and releases a hormone that regulates calcium levels and phosphate levels in the blood.

Pineal Gland: this term refers to the organ located in the third ventricle of the cerebrum. This organ converts nervous system messages into hormones. For instance, melatonin sends the message for sleep due to the sensing of darkness.

Pituitary Gland: this term refers to the organ that is attached to the hypothalamus which releases oxytocin and antidiuretic hormones, thyroid stimulating, gonadotropins, prolactin, and growth hormones.

Right Lymphatic Duct: this term refers to the duct or canal which gathers lymph from the right side and drains into the right subclavian near the right jugular and then adds it back into the blood stream.

Sebaceous Glands: this term refers to the sweat glands which are concentrated in the hands and feet. The hands and feet are most active in the environment and therefore have the thickest layers of skin and also have the most erosion of skin cells. Sebaceous glands in the integument release sebum which moistens the skin and is an antibacterial substance.

Spleen: this term refers to the organ located between the 6th and 11th ribs inferior to the diaphragm. The spleen stores iron, removes abnormal blood cells, and initiates the immune response. The spleen produces red blood cells in the fetus.

Stratum corneum: this term refers to the outermost layer of the skin.

Stratum Germinativum: this term refers to the deepest layer of skin which is divided into two parts: the stratum spinosum and the stratum basale. New cells are generated in this deepest layer.

Thymus: this term refers to the organ located behind the sternum in the anterior mediastinum, which produces the T cells or immune agents.

Thyroid Gland: this term refers to the organ that is located in the anterior of the neck and releases thyroxine and calcitonin.

Tonsils: this term refers to the organ which can trap bacteria and viruses. This organ located at the back of the throat and works to produce antibodies that fight disease.

The Muscular System

The back

The muscles of the back include: deltoid, erector spinae-spinalis, iliocostalis, longissimus, infraspinatus, interspinales, intertransversarii, latissimus dorsi, levator scapulae, levatores costarum, obliquus capitis inferior, obliquus capitis superior, rectus capitis posterior major, rectus capitis posterior minor; rhomboid major, rhomboid minor, serratus posterior inferior, serratus posterior superior, splenius capitis, splenius cervicis, supraspinatus, teres major, teres minor, transversospinalis-multifidus, rotators, semispinalis, and trapezius.

The head and neck

The muscles of the head and neck include: aryepiglotticus, auricularis, buccinators, constrictor of pharynx-inferior, middle, superior, corrugator supercilii, cricothyroid, depressor anguli oris, depressor labii inferioris, digastric, frontalis, genioglossus, geniohyoid, hyoglossus, inferior oblique, inferior rectus, intrinsic muscles of tongue, lateral cricoarytenoid, lateral pterygoid, lateral rectus, levator anguli oris, levator labii superioris, alaeque nasi, levator palpebrae superioris, levator veli palatine, longus capitis, longus colli, masseter, medial pterygoid, medial rectus, mentalis, uvulae, mylohyoid, nasalis, oblique arytenoid, obliquus capitis inferior, obliquus capitis superior, omohyoid, orbicularis oculi, orbicularis oris, palatoglossus, palatopharyngeus, platysma, posterior cricoarytenoid, procerus, rectus capitis anterior, anterior, lateralis, posterior major, posterior minor, risorius, salpingopharyngeus, scalenus anterior, scalenus medius, scalenus minimus; scalenus posterior, splenius capitis, splenius cervicis, stapedius, sternocleidomastoid, sternohyoid, styloglossus, stylohyoid, stylopharyngeus, superior oblique, superior rectus, temporalis, temporoparietalis, tensor tympani, tensor veli palatine, thyroarytenoid and vocalis, thyroepiglotticus, thyrohyoid, transverse arytenoid, major zygomaticus, and minor zygomaticus.

Types of muscles

The muscle types include the cardiac muscle, the skeletal muscles, and the smooth muscles. Cardiac is an involuntary, striated muscle found only in the heart. It is myogenic and stimulates its own contractions without nudges or any signals from the nervous system. Each cardiac muscle cell has an electric impulse built in that contract rhythmically all by itself. If this muscle is connected to other cardiac cells it will contract to stimulate the others in a synchronous rhythm. Skeletal is a striated muscle attached to the skeleton that works in sync with other skeletal muscles to move the body with contractions. Smooth muscles are non-striated muscles found in the walls and linings of organs.

Thorax

The muscles found in the thorax include the diaphragm; the intercostals external; the intercostals internal; the levatores costarum; the major and the minor pectoralis; the serratus anterior; the posterior inferior: the posterior superior; the subcostalis; and the transversus thoracis.

Important terms

Abdomen: this term refers to the cavity of the body located between the diaphragm and the pelvis.

Abduct: this term refers to progress away from the middle.

Adduct: this term refers to movement more toward the middle.

Adenology: this term refers to the study of the endocrine system in the body.

Alimentary Canal: this term refers to the digestive tract from the mouth to the anus.

Alveolus: this term refers to the small cavities found in the bronchioles of the lungs.

Ampulla: this term refers to a tube, duct or sac dilation.

Anastomosis: this term refers to the connection between vessels within the body.

Anatomy: this term refers to the study of the structure of an organism such as the human body.

Aneurysm: this term refers to a dilation of the wall of an artery that looks like a sac and is filled with blood.

Angiology: this term refers to the study of the circulatory system within the body.

Anterior Nares: this term refers to the external nasal openings in the nose.

Antrum: this term refers to a cavity within the body.

Aorta: this term refers to the arterial system or main artery within the body.

Apex: this term refers to the top or the pointed end at the top of an area.

Aponeurosis: this term refers to a tendon which is a fibrous tissue on muscles within the body.

Appendicular Skeleton: this term refers to the appendages or the bones of the arms and legs in the body.

Arteries: this term refers to the blood vessels which carry the blood away from the heart.

Arterioles: this term refers to the arteries ranging in size of about .2mm which connect to the capillary network of the circulatory system.

Articulation: this term refers to a joint where two bones make contact in such a way movement is possible.

Ascending Colon: this term refers to the large intestine on the right side of the abdomen within the body.

Atrium: this term refers to the chamber or cavity.

Autolysis: this term refers to the self-digestion of lysosomes. This process occurs when lysosomes enter the extra cellular fluid during decomposition to digest the body's tissue.

Axial Skeleton: this term refers to the 74 bones of the upright axis along with the 6 bones in the middle ear.

Bilateral: this term refers to the two sides of something.

Biopsy: this term refers to the extraction of tissue from tissues found in the body.

Bronchiole: this term refers to the smaller branches of the bronchus.

Bronchus: this term refers to one of the trachea branches found in the lungs.

Buccal Cavity: this term refers to the entrance to the oral cavity or the space between the teeth, gums and the lips in the mouth.

Calyx: this term refers to the cup-shaped division of the renal pelvis.

Capillary: this term refers to the blood and lymph vessels which connect arterioles with venules in the circulatory system.

Carpal: this term refers to the wrist and that which pertains to the wrist.

Caudal: this term refers to that which pertains to the tail.

Cecum: this term refers to the pocket at the end of the large intestine in the body.

Celiac: this term refers to that which relates to the abdomen in the body.

Cell Anatomy: this term refers to the parts of the cell including the nucleus. The nucleus contains communication openings so that it can send signals through the cellular components and the openings are called nuclear pores. Everything contained within the nucleus is called nucleoplasm. Cells contain chromosomes and genes which store genetic material.

Cephalic: this term refers to that which pertains to the head of the body.

Cervix: this term refers to the neck of the womb or any body part that resembles the shape of a neck.

Chromosomes: this term refers to the 46 chromosomes which are found in the human body. There are 23 chromosomes from the egg and 23 from the sperm.

Cilia: this term refers to the hair-like structures that move mucous and trapped particles away from the lungs.

Concha: this term refers to the external ear which derives its name because it is the part of the body shaped like a conch shell.

Condyle: this term refers to a rounded projection or ridge.

Cortex: this term refers to the outer covering of an internal organ.

Costa: this term refers to that which relates to the ribs within the body.

Crest: this term refers to a ridge or protrusion.

Cubital: this term refers to that which relates to the forearm within the body.

Cutaneous: this term refers to anything that concerns the skin.

Cytology: this term is derived from the Greek kytos meaning "container". It encompasses physiology, the composition, the life cycles, reproduction, and death of cells within the body.

Deferens: this term means to carry away.

Descending Colon: this term refers to the part of the large intestine on the left side of the abdomen within the body.

Distal: this term refers to the end or toward the end of a formation.

Diverticulum: this term refers to a small pouch, blisters, or bulges in the intestines which can fill up with debris and become infected from the debris that is not excreted from the body.

DNA: this abbreviation refers to the long spiraled molecule of DNA or deoxyribonucleic acid. Each ladder or spiraled molecule has a nitrogenous base which pairs off in specific ways and connects the sides together. The sides are alternating bands of sugar and phosphate.

Dorsal: this term refers to the posterior or the back side of the body.

Duodenum: this term refers to the part of the small intestine that is attached to the stomach.

Endocrine: this term refers to the system of the body that secretes into the blood or tissues rather than into a sac or duct.

Endothelium: this term refers to the lining of blood and lymphatic vessels within the body.

Epiphyses: this term refers to the long bone ends found in the body.

Epithelium: this term refers to the lining of glands, bowel, skin, and organs within the body.

Excision: this term refers to the whole removal of the tumorous tissue found in the body. An example of an excision is in a mastectomy.

Exocrine: this term refers to the system that secretes into a duct or sac in the body.

Exocytosis: this term refers to the body's process of secretion.

Externa Adventitia: this term refers to the blood vessel's outer coating or the lymph vessel's outer coating.

External: this term refers to the exterior or outside of something.

Fascia: this term refers to the connective tissue that is in the form of a sheet.

Fissure: this term refers to a furrow or channel.

Flagella: this term refers to the whip-like structures that move the sperm after it is activated within the vagina.

Foramen: this term refers to a hole in which a cord might run through. For example: the holes in the spinal column allow the spinal cord runs through their opening.

Fossa: this term refers to a concave or depression such as that of a socket found in the body.

Fovea: this term refers to a cavity found in the body.

Frontal Eminences: this term refers to the part of the forehead which is the farthest outward point above the eyebrows or hair found above the eyes.

Frontal Sinuses: this term refers to the hollows above the eyes in the forehead bones of the face.

Fundus: this term refers to the part of a hollow organ farthest from its inlet.

Gall Bladder: this term refers to the pear-shaped, sac like organ which stores bile. It is located under the liver.

Gastric: this term refers to anything which relates to the stomach in the body.

Genes: this term refers to the segments of DNA which control the movement of protein and determine the cell's function within the system. Genetic material is stored by DNA and this allows replication of the cell and the genetic material. The organic elements in the nucleic acids of DNA are carbon, oxygen, nitrogen and phosphorus. Ribosomes: this term refers to the manufacture of proteins from amino acids which attach to the endoplasmic reticulum. RNA (ribonucleic acid) and protein molecules make up the composition of ribosomes. Endoplasmic Reticulum: this term refers to the ER or the cellular membrane network which allows protein, carbohydrate and lipid synthesis, to be stored as substances within the cell without disturbing its cellular functions. It is the intracellular transport system of the body.

Germ Cells: this term refers to the reproductive cells called spermatozoa and oocytes which are not bacteria and are found within the body.

Glossal: this term refers to anything which relates to the tongue in the body.

Golgi: this term refers to the apparatus in the cell which is a part of the membrane that conducts and processes proteins to the plasma membrane, lysosomes, or endosomes. This apparatus functions as a central processing unit for the cell. This central processing unit controls all the incoming and the outgoing transportation of lipids.

Head: this term refers to the rounded portion which protrudes at the top of the skeletal system above a neck-like extension.

Hepar: this term refers to anything which relates to the liver or is hepatic in nature.

Histology: this term refers to the study of tissue at the microscopic level. Histology includes epithelium, endothelium, mesothelium, mesenchyme, and other tissues in the body.

Hyoid: this refers to the shape which forms the letter "u".

Ileum: this term refers to the part of the small intestine which is the third section of that organ.

Inferior: this term refers to anything in the lower area.

Inguinal: this term refers to that which relates to the groin.

Integumentary: this term refers to the cutis, derma, or skin. This system has two parts: the dermis and the epidermis. This is the system which has the sweat glands, sebaceous glands, touch corpuscles, and hair follicles.

Interstitial: this term refers to the small space between cells within the body.

Jejunum: this term refers to the second section of the small intestine within the body.

Joints: this refers to the points of connection between two or more bones within the body.

Labia: this term refers to the lips of the mouth.

Lacrimal: this term refers to anything which pertains or has to do with tears.

Lacuna: this term refers to the cavity or space in the body. One example of this is a space which holds bone cells.

Larynx: this term refers to the voice box located between the pharynx and trachea in the body.

Lateral: this term refers to that which is on the side or toward the side of the body.

Linear Guide: this term refers to a line drawn on the surface of the body to denote location of underlying structure(s) within.

Lipids: this term refers to the hydrocarbons which contain the organic compounds that ensure the health of the cells.

Liver: this term refers to the hepatic system containing the largest gland responsible to metabolize carbohydrates and protein. This system also is able to produce and secrete bile.

Lumen: this term refers to the central hole of a vessel or tube within the body.

Lungs: this term refers to the spongy organs located in the chest around the heart that is the main part of the respiratory system.

Lysosomes: this term refers to the digestive unit which contains different kinds of enzymes that breakdown proteins, nucleic acids, lipids, and carbohydrates. The substances produced from the breakdowns are then freed back into cytoplasm to form new substances. Lysosomes also play a large part in the body's immune system because they breakdown invading microbes that can harm the body.

Manubrium: this term refers to the upper structure of the sternum of the body.

Meatus: this is the general term for an opening in the body.

Medial: this term refers to the center or having location toward the middle.

Mediastinum: this term refers to the middle section between the lungs in the thorax of the body.

Medulla: this term refers to the marrow or the inside of an organ.

Membrane: this term refers to a layer or thin sheet of tissue in the body.

Mesenchyme: this term refers to the space-filling cells found in fat, bone, and muscles within the body.

Mesentery: this term refers to the part of the peritoneum that holds the intestine to the back of the abdomen within the body.

Mesial: this term refers to that which is in the middle or pertains to the median.

Mesothelium: this term refers to the lining of pleural, peritoneal, and pericardial spaces within the body.

Metabolism: this term refers to one of the functions of physiology which has to do with the biological energy or activeness of the body. Metabolism is defined in this formula: the basic Fuel + Oxygen = Carbon Dioxide + Water + Heat.

Microvilli: this term refers to the finger-like structures which absorb nutrients and other matter from extra cellular fluid.

Mitochondria: this term refers to the energy produced in a cell. This produces adenosine triphosphate (ATP) which requires both oxygen and carbon dioxide. Mitochondria have their own DNA and ribosomes so they replicate themselves within the cell. The highest energy is required in muscles where mitochondria are found in high numbers.

Mobility Structures: this refers to the cells of microvilli, cilia, and flagella.

Morphology: this term refers to a type of anatomy that studies the structure of an organism.

Myology: this term refers to the study of the muscular system within the body.

Nares: this term refers to the nostrils within the nose.

Nasal Septum: this term refers to the bone and the cartilage with divides the nose cavity into left and right halves. It normally conjoins with the hard palate forming the shape of the number 7.

Neurology: this term refers to the study of nerves and nervous system of the body.

Neurons: this term refers to the conduction cells in the nervous system of the body.

Nuchal: this term refers to that which relates to the nape of the neck.

Occiput: this term refers to the posterior or dorsal portion of the cephalon or skull.

Olecranon: this term refers to the elbow of the body.

Olfactory: this term refers to that which relates to the sense of smell.

Ophthalmic: this term refers to that which relates to the eyes.

Organelles: this term refers to a part of the cells found in the body.

Orifice: this term refers to an aperture.

Ossicles: this term refers to the small bones of the tympanum or ear drum.

Palate: this term refers to both the hard and the soft parts of the roof of the mouth.

Palpebrae: this term refers to the eyelids.

Pancreas: this term refers to the organ of the body located near the stomach which secretes enzyme-filled fluid for digestion and the hormone insulin and glucagon.

Parietal: this term refers to that which concerns the walls of a cavity or of an organ.

Parotid: this term refers to locations close to the ear. The parotid glands secrete saliva into the mouth.

Pathological Anatomy: this term refers to the study of tissues found in live patients, but can include those found through autopsy. Tissues are extracted through biopsy or excision. The American Board of Pathology issues certification in this branch of study. The only other primary certification is in Clinical Pathology.

Pectineal: this term refers to that which relates to the pubic bone in the body.

Pectoral: this term refers to that which relates to the chest or breast of the body.

Peripheral: this term refers to that which is on the outside surface.

Phalanges: this term refers to the bones within the toes and the fingers of the hands and feet.

Pharynx: this term refers to the upper throat above the esophagus and below the mouth which is located in the upper digestive tract.

Phrenic: this term refers to that which relates to the diaphragm of the body.

Placenta: this term refers to the lining in which the fetus is attached to the wall of the uterus in a pregnant woman's body.

Plasma: this term refers to the non-cellular, 92% water, clear, yellowish solution in which blood cells are suspended.

Popliteal: this term refers to the posterior of the knee.

Posterior: this term refers to the dorsal or behind.

Process: this term refers to the projection or outgrowth of tissue.

Pronate: this term refers to the position of palm downward; when the body is on its back, the position of the palms face downward and the body is said to be in a prone position.

Prostate Gland: this term refers to the male part which is located at the beginning of the urethra and ejaculates semen into the urethra during intercourse.

Protein Biosynthesis: this term refers to the protein conversion process where ribosomes synthesize proteins in the cytoplasm or the inner cellular fluid of the cell.

Protuberance: this term refers to a swelling or outgrowth.

Proximal: this term refers to that which relates to a location or position nearest to the center of the body.

Pyloric Sphincter: this term refers to the muscular hole between the duodenum and stomach. This comes from the Greek pyl = gate and orus = guard.

Ramus: this term means branch.

Regional Anatomy: this term refers to the study of one particular part of the body and incorporates all the system's functions and their interactions in that one part of the body. This includes the circulatory, muscular, skeletal, and all the interrelations studied at the same time as that part of the body.

Renal: this term refers to that which relates to the kidneys.

Rugae: this term describes wrinkly or a condition that is full of folds.

Sagittal: this term refers to up and down rather than side to side.

Salivary Glands: this term refers to the three pairs of glands which supply saliva: parotid, sublingual and submaxillary.

Sclera: this term refers to the hard, tough, white outer part of the eye which protects the eyeball.

Sesamoid Bones: this term refers to the sesame seed-shaped bones found on the end of tendons. These bones are small and flat and are responsible for helping with pressure leverages.

Sigmoid Colon: this term refers to the portion of the large intestine that extends downward from the iliac crest and which has an S-shaped appearance.

Sinus: this term refers to the cavities which have spongy space in the bone.

Sphincter: this term refers to a muscle which closes an opening in the body.

Spinous Process: this term refers to the spine or pointed projections located on the backbone.

Splanchnic: this term refers to the internal organ rather than framework surrounding the organ.

Stem Cells: this term refers to the cell study of animal and human diseased tissues in the study of histopathology. This typically is preformed on live patients, although autopsy is a major tool in medical information gathering of this science.

Superior: this term refers to a position above something.

Supernate: this term refers to the position of the palms upward or when the body is face down. The most natural position is when the palms are face up and the body is in the supine position.

Supraorbital Margin: this term refers to the ridge of bone located just below the eyebrow on the face.

Symphysis: this term refers to the growing together as in the case of fibrocartilaginous indicating the fusion of two bones.

Systemic Anatomy: this term refers to the body-wide study of a particular system such as the skeletal, nervous or circulatory systems. Each system is taken as a whole rather than in sections relating to the body.

Systems: this term refers to the structure responsible for the functional groups of the body.

Tendon: this term refers to the fibrous, elongated tissue which attaches muscles to bones in such a way that the two can work together.

Thorax: this term refers to the part of the body known as the chest or relating to the chest.

Tibia: this term refers to the bone of the shin in the leg.

Trachea: this term refers to the part of respiratory system that consists of a tube that runs from the larynx to the bronchi.

Transportation: this term refers to the diameter of the vascular system which responds to the chemical productions in response to the demands that the metabolism rates place upon the body.

Transverse Colon: this term refers to the second part of the large intestine which crosses the abdomen horizontally above the small intestine lying just below the liver.

Transverse: this term refers to the crosswise position of lying across the body's axis.

Trochanter: this term refers to a large, bony bump on the thigh bone known as the femur to which large muscles are attached.

Tunica Adventitia: this term refers to the outer layer of a blood or tubular vessel made of fibroelastic tissue within the body.

Tunica Intima: this term refers to the internal serous tissue layer of an artery within the body.

Tunica Media: this term refers to the middle, muscular layer of a blood or tubular vessel within the body.

Tunics: this term refers to one of the outer layers of a hollow organ or blood vessel.

Ureters: this term refers to the tubes which drain urine from the kidneys to the bladder within the body.

Urethra: this term refers to the tube which drains urine from the bladder outside of the body. In males, semen is ejaculated through this tube.

Uvula: this term refers to the soft tissue which hangs at the back of the throat in the body.

Valve: this term refers to the muscular structure which controls flow of fluid in one direction within the body.

Vas: this term refers to a duct or vessel within the body.

Vascular: this term refers to that which relates to the blood stream system or blood vessels within the body.

Vastus: this term indicates a great size.

Veins: this term refers to the blood vessels that carry blood to the heart within the body.

Ventral: this term refers to that which relates to the belly or anterior or front of the body.

Ventricle: this term refers to the cavity in the heart which pumps blood away from the heart.

Vermiform Appendix: this term refers to the part of the intestines which is worm-shaped and attached to the cecum known as the appendix.

Xiphoid: this term refers to that which is shaped like a sword.

Zygoma: this term refers to a yoke.

Practice Test

Arts

1. A will is an instrument for the ordered disposition of real and personal property that is to take effect upon death. Which of the following is a requirement for a will to take effect?
    a. The will has a codicil.
    b. The deceased was of legal age.
    c. There was intestacy on the part of the legatee.
    d. Both B: and C:

2. The Funeral Rule, which is enforced by the Federal Trade Commission (FTC), has many provisions. These include mandated disclosures and restrictive actions. At the very start of a face-to-face discussion with the public regarding the selection of funeral goods or services and/or the prices of them, the funeral director is required to give the consumer:
    a. The GPL for retention upon collection and signed receipt of the Consumer Protection Fee
    b. The price for each item the consumer requests on dated company letterhead
    c. The GPL for retention, and the casket and vault price list for reference only
    d. The casket price list and vault price list for retention, and the GPL for reference only

3. The person with the authority and duty of final disposition who may or may not have "actual" custody (physical possession) of the deceased at a particular moment is considered to have what kind of custody?
    a. Caveat emptor
    b. Constructive
    c. Consignment
    d. Endowment

4. An insolvent estate is an estate of a deceased person whose assets are insufficient to pay the estate's debts, taxes, and administrative expenses. It is the state statute that controls the priority of these claims. In most states, though, the priority of claims—from top priority to lowest—is ordered as follows:
    a. Taxes, funeral expenses, and medical bills
    b. Medical bills, taxes, and funeral expenses
    c. Funeral expenses, administration expenses, and taxes
    d. Administration expenses, funeral expenses, and taxes

5. A federal government agency created to promote consumer protection, encourage free and fair competition, and prevent what regulators determine to be anti-competitive business practices is called:
    a. FTC
    b. ICCFA
    c. OSHA
    d. NFDA

6. A wrongful act by a person for which damages can be sought by the injured party through a civil lawsuit is called a:
   a. Tort
   b. Mutilation
   c. Obstruction
   d. Replevin

7. The power of a government to impose what it considers reasonable restrictions and laws on its citizens for the maintenance of public safety, health, order, and welfare is called:
   a. Tort
   b. Police power
   c. Restrictive covenant
   d. Uniform probate code

8. Which of the following funeral rites is conducted without the presence of the casketed body?
   a. Entombment service
   b. Memorial service
   c. Graveside service
   d. Traditional or complete cremation service

9. A deceased veteran or reservist who was entitled to receive retired military pay qualifies to receive an American flag after the completion and submittal of the APPLICATION FOR UNITED STATES FLAG FOR BURIAL PURPOSES form, also known as:
   a. VA Form 21-530
   b. SSA-721
   c. VA form 90-2008
   d. VA form 40-1330

10. A portable stretcher used by both ambulances and funeral homes to move the injured or deceased that is considered to be the most important item for transferring remains from a house or an institution is called a:
   a. Cot
   b. Flexible stretcher
   c. Transfer vehicle
   d. Church truck

11. Which of the following accurately describe the purposes of a death certificate?
   i. Shows vital statistics and cause of death for medical or actuarial research
   ii. Is the legal permanent record of the deceased
   iii. Is the legal document issued by the proper government agency authorizing the transportation and/or disposition of human remains
   iv. Is the legal record that final disposition has occurred
   a. i , ii, and iv
   b. ii and iv
   c. i and ii
   d. All of the above

12. A typical funeral cortege would be arranged in the following order:
   a. Lead car, hearse, clergy, pallbearers, family cars/limo, and procession
   b. Lead car, hearse, pallbearers, clergy, family cars/limo, and procession
   c. Hearse, lead car, clergy, pallbearers, family cars/limo, and procession
   d. Lead car, clergy, pallbearers, hearse, family cars/limo, and procession

13. The entryway, foyer, or lobby to a funeral home or church is also called the:
   a. Narthex
   b. Nave
   c. Niche
   d. Sanctuary

14. In the Roman Catholic faith, an anointing ceremony by a priest for the seriously ill to bring healing or for those who are dying to prepare their souls for eternity is called:
   a. Paschal Candle Service
   b. Sacrament of the Sick
   c. Rosary Service
   d. Rosary Beads

15. The name for the sanctified elements of Holy Communion that comprise the essential rudiments for liturgical worship is:
   a. Paschal Candle
   b. Communion Paten
   c. Eucharist
   d. Trisagion

16. Which of the following statements concerning the merchandise pricing strategy known as the Declining Price Structure Model is correct?
   a. Creates a lower margin on the less expensive caskets
   b. Creates a lower margin on the most expensive caskets
   c. Encourages the consumer to buy better merchandise since the CVI improves with higher-priced caskets
   d. Both b and c

17. A casket constructed of various tree species such as salix, poplar, or cottonwood is called:
   a. Single hinged panel
   b. Wood veneer
   c. Selected hardwood
   d. Pine box

18. There are various types of casket interior styles. In one style, the lining material is placed on a metal form. Weights are added, and the material is then steamed and attached to an upholstery or backing. This interior style is known as:
   a. Masselin
   b. Crushed
   c. Extendover
   d. Tufted

19. Caskets use various lining materials. One material is a thin, crinkled cloth made of silk, cotton, rayon, or wool called:
    a. Crepe
    b. Satin
    c. Velvet
    d. Linen

20. A monument that is erected to the memory of the dead but may not serve as the physical resting place for the deceased is called a:
    a. Cenotaph
    b. Crypt
    c. Epitaph
    d. Columbarium

21. What are the two broad classifications of metal?
    a. Bronze and copper
    b. Stainless steel and steel
    c. Galvanized steel and steel
    d. Ferrous and non-ferrous

22. What are the four component parts of casket handles?
    a. Arm, bar, shell, and tip
    b. Lug, rim, shell, and tip
    c. Lug, arm, bar, and shell
    d. Lug, arm, bar, and tip

23. A metal alloy of steel chromium and sometimes nickel that has a noted ability to resist rust is:
    a. Copper
    b. Bronze
    c. Steel
    d. Stainless steel

24. During the arrangement conference, the process whereby the funeral director listens to the client with undivided attention and maintains eye contact to watch the client's non-verbal body language (such as facial expressions) is called:
    a. Adaptive
    b. Paraphrasing
    c. Attending
    d. Summarizing

25. In her book On Death and Dying (1969), Elisabeth Kubler-Ross identifies and describes the stages of dying. In order, these stages are:
    a. Accept, express, adjust, and reinvest
    b. Numbness, yearning, disorganization and despair, and re-organization
    c. Shock, awareness of loss, conservation-withdrawal, and healing and renewal
    d. Denial, anger, bargaining, depression, and acceptance

26. The grieving and adaptation to living after the loss of a loved one is called:
    a. Mourning
    b. Bereavement
    c. Thanatology
    d. Grief

27. The common patterns and range of feelings and behaviors people exhibit after the loss of a loved one is called:
    a. Grief syndrome
    b. Guilt
    c. Shame
    d. Attachment theory

28. An expression of frustration and helplessness, during grief it is often deflected onto doctors, funeral directors, and other individuals. This expression is usually in the form of:
    a. Grief
    b. Guilt
    c. Anger
    d. Mourning

29. Grief that is excessive, does not come to a satisfactory conclusion, and is accompanied by the individual's awareness of their inability to resolve the bereavement process is called:
    a. Masked grief
    b. Delayed grief
    c. Chronic grief
    d. Exaggerated grief

30. To communicate with those who are mourning the recent loss of a loved one to facilitate the bereavement process and help them move through the stages of grief is called:
    a. At need counseling
    b. Grief therapy
    c. Grief counseling
    d. Both a and b

31. A trocar is a hollow tube used during the embalming process to inject fluids and drain excess fluids that was patented in 1868 by:
    a. Dr. William Harvey
    b. Samuel Rogers
    c. Gabriel Clauderus
    d. James A. Gray

32. Which of the following are the two entities worshipped in the Egyptian culture?
    a. Pagan and Natron
    b. Children Of Horus and canopic jars
    c. The Kher-heb and Libitinarius
    d. The sun and the cult of Osiris

33. In 1666, an act was passed in England's Parliament that instituted a monetary penalty for the use of commonly imported linen in coffin linings. Instead, the shroud had to be made of a linen substitute made in England (except in cases where the death was caused by the plague). This product was:
   a. Velvet
   b. Masselin
   c. Satin
   d. Wool

34. A single household that consists of one man, one woman, and their children (if they have any) is known as a:
   a. Nuclear family
   b. Extended(joint) family
   c. Modified extended family
   d. Blended family

35. Which type of family structure may be more receptive to an immediate cremation or a memorial service with a memory board of photos and a DVD made by the funeral director or the family?
   a. Extended (joint) family
   b. Bureaucratization family
   c. Nuclear family
   d. Demographic family

36. The science that studies various social groups and how individuals behave and relate to each other as a group to other social groups that can influence funeral service disposition arrangements is:
   a. Funeralization
   b. Ethnocentrism
   c. Pathology
   d. Sociology

37. The mobility of society today is a change in our culture that has had an effect on funeral service arrangements. The trend for people to move away from where they were born and raised and relocate to a new area for work or climate is called:
   a. Enculturation
   b. Ethnocentrism
   c. Social stratification
   d. Neo-localism

38. An assignment is a transfer of legal rights from one person (party) to another. The party to whom the assignment is made is called the:
   a. Assignor
   b. Beneficiary
   c. Consignee
   d. Assignee

39. The transfer of possession, but not title, of personal property such as rings or jewelry worn by the deceased from a family to a funeral director is called:
    a. Consignee
    b. Bailment
    c. Blank endorsement
    d. Acceptance

40. The person who executes a promissory note is called the:
    a. Maker
    b. Payee
    c. Drawee
    d. Drawer

41. Another name for the income statement that reports the profitability of a business is called:
    a. Statement of operations
    b. Balance sheet
    c. Statement of financial position
    d. Trial balance

42. The amount by which a business's current assets exceed liabilities, defined as the operating liquidity of a business, is also known as:
    a. Statement of operations
    b. Working capital
    c. Proving cash
    d. Useful life

43. A federal act that requires employers to withhold a portion of employee wages and pay them to the government trust fund that provides retirement benefits is called:
    a. Federal Income Tax Withholding
    b. Federal Unemployment Tax Act
    c. W-2
    d. Federal Insurance Contributions Act

44. A written promise from a client to pay a specific amount of money to a business on a specific, agreed-upon future date is called:
    a. Federal Income Tax Withholding
    b. Maker
    c. Note receivable
    d. Blank endorsement

45. Which of the following would be considered a data storage medium?
    a. Scanner
    b. Compact disc
    c. Jump drive
    d. Both b and c

46. When selecting a computer system that will be used for data processing, the preliminary key points to consider are:
    a. Viruses and spam
    b. Microsoft and Apple
    c. Needs and wants, software and hardware
    d. Wi-Fi and Internet

47. The "Two Factor Theory" is the psychological theory that peoples' motivation in the workplace is the result of multiple factors that influence their satisfaction or dissatisfaction. The theory was developed by:
    a. Abraham Maslow
    b. Douglas McGregor
    c. Frederick Herzberg
    d. Both a and b

48. Federal legislation that was designed to prohibit job discrimination on the basis of race, religion, color, national origin, and sex is called:
    a. Age Discrimination Employment Act
    b. Occupational Safety and Health Act
    c. Immigration Reform and Control Act
    d. Equal Employment Opportunity Act

49. The legal principle by which precedents are established by prior decisions made by the court that also serves to provide insight into the potential outcome of similar cases is called:
    a. Statute of Limitations
    b. Statutes
    c. Equal Employment Opportunity Act
    d. Stare Decisis

50. The gauge that represents a business's financial leverage, is determined by dividing the business's total liabilities by stockholders' equity, and also represents how much funding has been borrowed to finance the business is called:
    a. Current ratio
    b. Debt equity
    c. Book value
    d. Economic order quantity

51. There are three main factors that influence the grieving process. They are psychological, sociological, and:
    a. External
    b. Internal
    c. Physiological
    d. Illogical

52. Which of the following statements is true?
    a. All Native American tribes believe that birth is more sacred than death
    b. All Native American tribes believe the body is simply a shell that's left
    c. Some Native American tribes believe in an afterlife, and some don't
    d. All of the above statements are true

53. When a society believes that nothing is lost in death and that people can take things with them, this belief is known as which of the following?
    a. Death defiance
    b. Death denial
    c. Death acceptance
    d. Death reward

54 The Jewish religion executes many rituals when someone dies. The preparation of the body for burial is called:
    a. Shiva
    b. Chevra kadisha
    c. Yahrzeit
    d. Tahara

55. There are two types of violent death. One is homicide. What is the other?
    a. Suicide
    b. Terminal illness
    c. Premature death
    d. A body that is not recovered

56. Complicated grief may occur when socially unspeakable circumstances are present. An example of this might be which of the following?
    a. Abortion
    b. Death of a married lover
    c. Death of an abusive parent
    d. All of the above

57. The four items that affect an individual's views on death are religion, family, culture, and:
    a. Gender
    b. Race
    c. Tradition
    d. Financial status

58. When working with a family, you notice that one person seems to be struggling. When you approach this person, he says with strong hesitation, "I'm fine." This is an example of which type of nonverbal communication?
    a. Facial expression
    b. Paralanguage
    c. Proxemics
    d. Body position

59. When a funeral home offers various types of assistance for the grieving after the funeral services are over, it is known as:
    a. Aftercare
    b. Preneed
    c. The arrangement conference
    d. Complicated grief

60. A funeral director can help a family with their grief by doing which of the following?
   a. Tell them they don't need to write the obituary
   b. Offer to give the eulogy so a family member doesn't have to
   c. Explain that they don't need to go to the cemetery
   d. Allow them to bring in items from a collection their loved one had

61. Which of the following is true of Elisabeth Kubler-Ross's five stages of grief?
   a. They do not always occur in order
   b. A grieving person usually completes them in about six months
   c. Each one takes about the same amount of time
   d. When people try to make a deal with God, it is called "denial"

62. Which of the following should an adult do when a child is grieving?
   a. Wait to tell them about the death until it is absolutely necessary
   b. Keep them from going to the cemetery
   c. Let them participate in the funeral if they want to
   d. Encourage them not to talk about it to other people

63. A funeral director can help family members by acknowledging their grief. Of the following family members, which person's grief is usually acknowledged the least by society?
   a. A spouse
   b. A sibling
   c. A parent
   d. A child

64. Which of the following must be notified when you are planning a service that includes visiting hours, a funeral, and a burial?
   a. The officiating person and the cemetery
   b. The burial vault company and the cemetery
   c. The officiating person only
   d. The officiating person, the cemetery, and the burial vault company

65. When entering a Catholic church for a Mass of Christian Burial, the casket is covered with which of the following?
   a. A pall
   b. A veil
   c. A flag
   d. A blanket

66. Which of the following is the best course of action for a funeral director when a funeral will be held at a place of worship where he/she has never been?
   a. Figure out how the service will be handled when he/she arrives
   b. Call the officiating person to get specific information about the handling of the service
   c. Check to see if there is any helpful information online
   d. Let a family member direct the service

67. Most crematories require the body of the deceased to be in a rigid container for the cremation process. Which of the following does NOT meet the definition of most crematories of a rigid container?
    a. The deceased is in a mahogany casket
    b. The deceased is wrapped in a sheet
    c. The deceased is on a flat board
    d. The deceased is in a cardboard box

68. A deceased veteran must meet which of the following criteria in order to be eligible for military honors?
    a. Have an "honorable" discharge
    b. Obtained the rank of sergeant or higher
    c. Died during wartime
    d. Have a discharge other than "dishonorable"

69. Which of the following is the most important part of the arrangement conference?
    a. Getting the death certificate information
    b. Listening carefully
    c. Writing the obituary
    d. Explaining the costs

70. Most green cemeteries adhere to which of the following rules?
    a. The body cannot be dressed
    b. The body cannot be in a casket
    c. The body must be placed into a concrete vault
    d. The body cannot be embalmed

71. Which of the following statements is true about shipping human remains via common carrier within the United States?
    a. They have to be embalmed
    b. They have to be sent prepaid
    c. They must be in a casket
    d. They must be accompanied with a burial/transit permit

72. During an arrangement conference, a family member says he would like to bring in a peanut butter jar for his father's cremated remains. What is the best way for the funeral director to respond?
    a. Tell him that this is not allowed by law
    b. Explain that the crematory will not allow it
    c. Explain that if the jar is not large enough, the rest of the remains will have to be put into another container
    d. Suggest that the family purchase an urn on which a picture of a peanut butter jar can be engraved

73. When you accept jewelry from the next of kin to place on the deceased, you become known as what?
   a. Bailee
   b. Mediator
   c. Conservator
   d. Codicil

74. If a funeral director takes a picture of a deceased without the permission of the next of kin, which of the following could he/she be guilty of?
   a. Libel
   b. Immunity
   c. Grand larceny
   d. Habeas corpus

75. If a woman deposits money in a preneed burial account at her local bank, the bank assumes which of the following roles?
   a. Assignee
   b. Devisee
   c. Fiduciary
   d. Distributee

76. When the funeral director and the purchaser of funeral services sign an agreement, this is known as which of the following?
   a. Employment contract
   b. Quid pro quo
   c. Confidentiality agreement
   d. Limited liability

77. When a beneficiary brings in a life insurance policy to be used as payment for the funeral services, he/she signs a form. What is this form called?
   a. An assignment
   b A consideration
   c. A comfort letter
   d. A mediation

78. When a funeral director begins talking to another director about purchasing his/her funeral home, the potential purchaser will probably be asked to sign which of the following types of agreements?
   a. Collateral agreement
   b. Confidentiality agreement
   c. Consideration agreement
   d. Collective agreement

79. In most states, all of the following people can observe the embalming process EXCEPT which of the following?
   a. The attending physician
   b. Nonparticipating embalmers
   c. A family member of the deceased
   d. The embalmer's non-licensed spouse

80. Which of the following individuals can sign the appropriate forms to authorize the cremation of a body?
   a. An ex-spouse
   b. A medical doctor
   c. An agent assigned by the deceased in applicable states
   d. The deceased's clergyman

81. When making funeral arrangements, when must the funeral director give the customer a copy of the General Price List (GPL)?
   a. As soon as the customer sits down
   b. After taking all the information for the death certificate
   c. Before selecting the casket
   d. When any mention of prices or costs is brought up

82. John Doe dies and does not leave a surviving wife. He does, however, have nine children, and some of them are expressing a desire to have his body cremated. In a state that requires the cremation process to be authorized by at least 60 percent of the children, how many must sign the authorization form?
   a. Three
   b. Five
   c. Six
   d. Seven

83. Someone calls the funeral home and asks about your prices. According to the Funeral Rule, which of the following must you do?
   a. Read your entire General Price List to them
   b. Send them a copy of your General Price List
   c. Explain that if they come to the funeral home you will give them pricing information
   d. Send them a copy of your General Price List only if you wish to

84. Embalming is necessary in which of the following situations?
   a. When the family chooses a direct burial
   b. When the FTC Funeral Rule requires it
   c. When the deceased will be shipped out of town
   d. When the family requests it

85. When someone pays a deposit or the entire amount for a preplanned funeral, all of the following can be done with the funds EXCEPT:
   a. The entire amount can be deposited into the funeral home's bank account
   b. The funds can be deposited into an account at the local bank
   c. The funds can be deposited into the state funeral director association's trust fund
   d. In some states, the funds can be used for a life insurance policy for the deceased

86. When funds have been prepaid for someone who is on Medicaid, they are deposited into an irrevocable account. If the funds in the account exceed the amount of the services provided when the death occurs, what happens to the leftover amount?
    a. It is returned to the next of kin in a personal check made out to him or her
    b. It must be sent to the Medicaid office
    c. The funeral home can keep the entire amount
    d. The institution where the money was deposited keeps it

87. It is illegal to do which of the following?
    a. Show pictures of caskets instead of displaying actual caskets
    b. Display caskets in order of price
    c. Display all the wooden caskets together and all the metal caskets together
    d. Display a casket without its price

88. Caskets can be displayed in a selection room or in a catalog of photos. Which of the following is another way they can be displayed?
    a. The Casket Price List
    b. The General Price List
    c. Photos on a computer
    d. The Burial Container Price List

89. What is the most important part of displaying burial vaults?
    a. Having a full-size vault in your selection room
    b. Being able to explain the characteristics and advantages of each vault
    c. Having a cross section of a vault
    d. Showing pictures of vaults

90. Which of the following is an example of passive marketing?
    a. Having products or their photos displayed and allowing the customer to initiate discussion about them
    b. Showing customers the caskets on display in the selection room
    c. Showing pictures of vaults to customers
    d. Giving the customer a GPL

91. Which of the following items should be displayed since they can easily be personalized at any funeral home with a computer?
    a. Prayer cards/memorial folder with a choice of prayers or poems and the option to add the deceased's photo
    b. Cremation jewelry with names and dates
    c. Monuments
    d. Urns with photos

92. Usually, merchandising is done with products. Which of the following is an effective way to merchandise a funeral home's services?
    a. The General Price List
    b. An informational brochure
    c. A display of urns
    d. Pictures of monuments

93. A software program made specifically for funeral homes could help you do which of the following?
  a. Send an email to your staff about an upcoming event
  b. Print out your vehicle registration cards
  c. Build a website
  d. Design and print prayer cards or funeral folders

94. Which of the following would most likely be used to keep track of funeral home expenses?
  a. A word processing computer program
  b. An accounting computer program
  c. A calculator
  d. An email program

95. Which of the following is a liability?
  a. The funeral home
  b. Vehicles
  c. Payroll
  d. Office equipment

96. Depreciation can be claimed on which of the following?
  a. Health insurance
  b. Vehicles
  c. Legal expenses
  d. Payroll

97. When you record a payment made for a funeral, it will decrease the amount associated with which of the following?
  a. Accounts payable
  b. Accounts receivable
  c. Expenses
  d. Assets

98. Which of the following is the best reason to have a website for your funeral home?
  a. It will allow you to post pictures of your children
  b. It will provide helpful information to anyone who visits it
  c. It will help with your funeral home accounting procedures
  d. You can send email to your staff and customers from it

99. When a family brings in an actual picture of the deceased to be placed on the memorial folders or prayer cards, you should use which of the following devices with your computer to get the best result?
  a. A scanner
  b. A cell phone
  c. A digital camera
  d. A memory card

100. A trial balance will help a business owner do which of the following?
    a. Keep track of inventory
    b. Help with vehicle maintenance
    c. Show profits and losses
    d. Ensure accurate payroll

Science

1. What group of chemicals is used in funeral preparations in extreme cases, such as bodies with edema or ones exhibiting advanced decomposition?
    a. Low index fluids
    b. Humectants
    c. High index fluids
    d. Water conditioning

2. When is the correct time to inject tissue builder with a hypodermic syringe?
    a. After embalming
    b. Before closing the mouth
    c. After disinfecting
    d. Before embalming

3. A written record and sketch diagram of the condition of the body upon arrival to the funeral home, the method of embalming, treatments, the times at which the body arrived and preparations were completed, and the license numbers of the embalmers and assistants is called the:
    a. Putrefaction case report
    b. Sanitation case report
    c. Decomposition case report
    d. Embalming case report

4. Admittance to the preparation room while a deceased is present should only be granted to:
    a. Licensees
    b. Those authorized by the family or the state
    c. Pre-need counselors
    d. Both a and b

5. The difference between the potential pressure reading and the actual pressure reading indicates the:
    a. Vacuum pressure
    b. Rate of flow
    c. Differential pressure
    d. Both b and c

6. A blunt instrument used for tissue dissection and for determining the location and elevation of arteries and veins that is especially useful after the initial incision to locate the carotid artery and jugular vein is made is called.
    a. Bistoury knife
    b. Hemostat
    c. Aneurism needle
    d. Forceps

7. The study of death and dying that places an emphasis on the psychological and social aspects is called:
    a. Psychology
    b. Psychiatry
    c. Pathology
    d. Thanatology

8. The process by which blood settles or pools within the vessels to the dependent or lowest parts of the body as a result of gravitational movement is called:
    a. Agonal hypostasis
    b. Hemolysis
    c. Intermittent drainage
    d. Agonal mortis

9. The chemical reaction in which the chemical bonds of a substance are split by the addition or taking up of water that is also the single most important factor in the initiation of decomposition is called:
    a. Hemolysis
    b. Hydrolysis
    c. Hematemesis
    d. Fermentation

10. Rigor mortis can be broken down by which of the following physical methods?
    a. Flexing or bending
    b. Rotating
    c. Massaging the joints
    d. All of the above

11. The Centers for Disease Control concluded that funeral directors had an elevated risk of contracting a variety of bloodborne and airborne pathogens as a result of their contact with dead human bodies, and found that the most frequently reported diseases by funeral directors included:
    a. Hematoma
    b. Staphylococcal infection
    c. Cutaneous tuberculosis
    d. Both b and c

12. The ventilation of a prep room is measured using the number of air exchanges per hour. This is calculated by taking the total square footage of the room and then determining the size of the air handler or fan needed to move the air out and replace it in a given amount of time. According to Robert Mayer author of Embalming: History, Theory & Practice; the air exchange rate for a preparation room should be between _____ and _____ per hour.
   a. 5 – 8
   b. 5 – 10
   c. 20 – 30
   d. 12 – 20

13. There are approximately six devices that can be used to inject arterial solution. Which of the following is NOT a device historically used during embalming?
   a. Bulb syringe
   b. Gravity bottle
   c. Centrifugal pump
   d. Hand pump

14. Another term used to describe the front, or anterior, of the body is:
   a. Dorsal
   b. Anatomical position
   c. Medial
   d. Ventral

15. A type of suture used to close incisions so that the ligature remains entirely under the epidermis is called:
   a. Basket weave suture
   b. Intradermal suture
   c. Bridge stitch
   d. Loop stitch

16. The natural facial marking that is a small convex distinction found lateral to the end of the line of closure of the mouth is called the:
   a. Frontal eminences
   b. Angulus oris sulcus
   c. Frontal process of the maxilla
   d. Angulus oris eminence

17. To ensure a successful application, an embalmer will usually apply surface mortuary wax to a deceased:
   a. Approximately three to six hours after embalming
   b. Immediately after embalming is completed
   c. Before embalming is started
   d. Not less than twenty-four hours after embalming

18. The most common of the basic linear forms of facial profiles is called:
   a. Vertical balanced profile
   b. Convex profile
   c. Concave profile
   d. Horizontally balanced profile

19. A type of incomplete fracture in which the bone may become bent or broken but does not go through the skin is called a:
   a. Compound fracture
   b. Third degree fracture
   c. Open fracture
   d. Closed or greenstick fracture

20. A suture made around a circular opening or puncture that closes the margins when it is pulled is called a:
   a. Basket weave suture
   b. Purse suture
   c. Bridge suture
   d. Whip suture

21. Cosmetics can be classified by their ability to allow light to pass through them. The type that does not allow light to pass through and is considered a concealing cosmetic is:
   a. Translucent
   b. Transparent
   c. Opaque
   d. Aerosol

22. There are seven basic shapes that describe the form of a head when observed from the front. The most common is where the cheekbones are wider than the cranium and the cranium is a little wider than the lower jaw. This shape is called:
   a. Diamond
   b. Oval
   c. Round
   d. Oblong

23. The groove at the end of the line of closure that forms between the two mucous membranes when the mouth is closed is called the:
   a. Weather line
   b. Medial lobe
   c. Angulus oris eminence
   d. Angulus oris sulcus

24. The name of the bones that create the superior portion of the sides and the back of the cranium and account for the posterior two-thirds of the roof of the cranium is:
   a. Parietal
   b. Occipital
   c. Temporal
   d. Zygomatic

25. The muscle that is the strongest chewing muscle of mastication and the one that assists in side-to-side movement of the mandible is the:
   a. Temporal
   b. Temporalis
   c. Levator labii superioris
   d. Corrugators

26. The physiognomic descriptions of facial markings include those that are natural at birth and those that are acquired over time as a result of the repeated use of muscles and age. Which of the following is a facial marking acquired over time?
    a. Nasal sulcus
    b. Nasolabial fold
    c. Philtrum
    d. Nasolabial sulcus

27. Bacteria are separated into three general groups according to their cellular shape. Which of the following is the term used to describe a bacterium that is rod-shaped or cylindrical?
    a. Vibrio
    b. Coccus
    c. Spiral
    d. Bacillus

28. A type of bacterium that is known as a tissue gas and can be transmitted from one deceased person to another as a result of improper disinfection of the trocar between uses is:
    a. Streptococcus pyogenes
    b. Clostridium perfringens
    c. Clostridium tetani
    d. Staphylococcus aureus

29. The study of bacteria—specifically its size, shape, and physical features—is:
    a. Mycology
    b. Morphology
    c. Virology
    d. Immunology

30. There are several physical methods to control microorganisms. Which of the following physical methods is generally accepted as the least bactericidal?
    a. Dry heat
    b. Moist heat
    c. Autoclave
    d. Cold

31. Which of the following modes of transmission of infections is a form of direct transmission?
    a. Food
    b. Fomite
    c. Droplet
    d. Milk

32. The term for the condition in which excess blood is localized or pooled in an area that is not able to allow for the normal drainage movement of blood as a result of a disease is called:
    a. Thrombosis
    b. Passive hyperemia
    c. Active hyperemia
    d. Embolism

33. Hemorrhages can be classified based on where they actually occur. When there is bleeding inside the pleural cavity, it is known as a(n):
    a. Epistaxis
    b. Hemopericardium
    c. Hemoperitoneum
    d. Hemothorax

34. When hemolysis of red blood cells occurs in a corpse and the result is post-mortem stain, the coloring matter pigment made from inside the body is referred to as:
    a. Endogenous
    b. Fomite
    c. Atrophy
    d. Exogenous

35. A common lesion such as a blister that forms an elevation on the skin and contains fluid is a:
    a. Furuncle
    b. Vesicle
    c. Ulcer
    d. Carbuncle

36. A condition in which there is a decrease in the number of white blood cells (leukocytes) that help fight disease circulating in the blood is:
    a. Hemophilia
    b. Leukemia
    c. Polycythemia
    d. Leucopenia

37. A viral infection characterized by inflammation of the liver that is likely transmitted by contaminated body fluids and is a concern to embalmers is:
    a. Hemophilia
    b. Hepatitis A
    c. Hemorrhage
    d. Hepatitis B

38. Neurotropic diseases can be caused by infectious diseases that affect the nervous system and often create inflammation. The most specific term for the disease condition in which inflammation and swelling of the brain occurs is:
    a. Encephalitis
    b. Meningitis
    c. Myelitis
    d. Poliomyelitis

39. Which of the following is the main organ of the integumentary system?
    a. Pleural cavity
    b. Heart
    c. Skin
    d. Epididymis

40. The molecular movement of matter from an area of greater concentration to an area of lower concentration is:
   a. Hydrolysis
   b. Saturation
   c. Diffusion
   d. Compound

41. When a solution has all the solvent it can hold, this condition is known as:
   a. Saturation
   b. Sublimation
   c. Inflammation
   d. Binary fission

42. The decomposition of human remains is a chemical change in which matter is broken down into smaller types of matter. The most significant process related to this change is:
   a. Vaporization
   b. Diffusion
   c. Adsorption
   d. Hydrolysis

43. There are four major types of preservatives used in embalming fluids. One is formaldehyde. The other three are:
   a. Aldehydes, alcohols, and phenols
   b. Sterols, phenols, and alcohol
   c. Sterols, lipids, and alcohol
   d. Aldehydes, sterols, and phenols

44. The major source of formaldehyde in aqueous solution for human preservation purposes contains ____ percent HCHO gas by weight and ____ percent HCHO gas by volume in a compound commonly known as formalin.
   a. 40; 37
   b. 37; 40
   c. 37; 30
   d. 40; 27

45. Phalanges is the name used to classify bones in the distal portion of the:
   a. Hand
   b. Elbow
   c. Toes
   d. Both a and c

46. The hip contains a pair of coxal bones, and is made of three fused bones collectively known as:
   a. The patella
   b. The pelvic girdle
   c. The phalanges
   d. The circle of Willis

47. Which of the following correctly describes the amount of movement associated with a synarthrosis articulation?
   a. Not moveable
   b. Somewhat moveable
   c. Extremely moveable
   d. None of the above; synarthrosis does not refer to articulation

48. In order to study the human body, certain imaginary lines or planes are used to cut the body into different parts. The plane that divides the body into two equal and symmetrical halves is the:
   a. Median plane
   b. Coronal plane
   c. Transverse plane
   d. Both b and c

49. The branch of anatomy that studies how disease affects the structure and function of the body is:
   a. Regional anatomy
   b. Gross anatomy
   c. Pathological anatomy
   d. Systemic anatomy

50. The chemical secretions given off by the endocrine glands are called:
   a. Hormones
   b. Red blood cells
   c. White blood cells
   d. Bile

51. Which of the following is one of the main arteries commonly used in embalming?
   a. Iliac
   b. Ulnar
   c. Femoral
   d. Aorta

52. In cases where it is necessary to use an electric spatula, it must always be used with which of the following?
   a. Water
   b. Massage cream
   c. Soap
   d. Nothing

53. To calculate the number of ounces of fluid to use per gallon (128 ounces) of water for a 2 percent solution, which of the following formulas would you use?
   a. 2 x the index of the fluid ÷ 128
   b. 2 x 128 ÷ the index of the fluid
   c. The index of the fluid ÷ 128
   d. The index of the fluid x 128

54. Using intermittent drainage during embalming will do which of the following?
    a. Decrease saturation in the tissues
    b. Create clots
    c. Make aspirating the organs unnecessary
    d. Provide better distribution of the fluid

55. When embalming autopsied remains, which of the following arteries are not typically used for injection?
    a. Left and right iliac
    b. Left and right carotid
    c. Left and right jugular
    d. Left and right subclavian

56. When corneas have been donated, which of the following must be done?
    a. Remove the materials left by the tissue bank in the eye socket and discard
    b. Place an eye cap over the materials left in the eye socket by the tissue bank
    c. Carefully clean the outside of the eye and glue the eyelids to prevent any leakage only
    d. Excise any tissue remaining in the eye socket

57. There are four guides used in trocar aspiration. They serve to access the heart, cecum, urinary bladder, and:
    a. Lungs
    b. Liver
    c. Stomach
    d. Kidneys

58. Inexpert tests for death include which of the following?
    a. A ligature tied around a finger
    b. A small amount of ammonia injected subcutaneously
    c. Listening for respiration or a heartbeat with an ear over the chest
    d. All of the above

59. In cases where a body will not be embalmed, which of the following must be done for a private viewing or identification of the body?
    a. Closing the mouth and eyes
    b. Injection of a pre-injection fluid
    c. Cavity treatment
    d. Surface embalming

60. When embalming babies, which of the following parts of the process is the same as the one used for adults?
    a. Use of the needle injector for the mouth closure
    b. Positioning of both hands over the body
    c. Use of the same type of arterial fluids
    d. Use of the ascending aorta as an injection site

61. Autopsies can be done on the complete torso and cranium, and on which of the following?
    a. Thorax
    b. Arms
    c. Legs
    d. Neck

62. The four categories of embalming are cavity, arterial, hypodermic, and:
    a. Co-injection
    b. Autopsy
    c. Surface
    d. Pre-injection

63. Which of the following chemical fluids is used to prevent dehydration and maintain tissue moisture?
    a. Dyes
    b. Cavity chemicals
    c. Hardening compounds
    d. Humectants

64. Hypodermic injection is used in which of the following situations?
    a. Every embalming procedure
    b. Only with infants or children
    c. Only in cases with trauma
    d. When any tissue shows no signs of preservation

65. Which of the following is the study of facial proportions?
    a. Physiognomy
    b. Physiology
    c. Restorative art
    d. Facial positioning

66. How are the eyelids placed in a correct eye closure?
    a. They meet in the middle
    b. The top lid meets the bottom lid two-thirds of the way down the eye
    c. The top lid closes all the way down over the eye to overlap the bottom lid
    d. The top lid closes all the way down over the eye to meet the bottom lid

67. Before restoration can be done, what condition must be met?
    a. Affected tissue must be firm and moist
    b. Tissue must be firm and dry
    c. Tissue must be soft and dry
    d. Tissue must be soft and moist

68. Which of the following is a natural facial marking?
    a. Dimples
    b. Nasolabial sulcus
    c. Optic facial sulci
    d. Cords of the neck

69. Which of the following are types of facial profiles?
    a. Vertical and horizontal
    b. Convex, concave, and horizontal
    c. Convex, vertical, and horizontal
    d. Convex, concave, and vertical

70. Becoming proficient in restoring a deceased body is associated with which of the following benefits?
    a. It allows family members to get rid of a mental image of what the trauma may have done
    b. It gives people a chance to say a final farewell with appropriate closure
    c. It exceeds people's expectations when they knew the circumstances of a traumatic death
    d. All of the above

71. If there is not enough time or resources to do an adequate hair restoration, which of the following may be done?
    a. Leave it as is and give an explanation to the family
    b. Use a scarf for a woman and a similar head bandage for a man
    c. Start the procedure and explain to the family that you didn't have time, but will complete it later
    d. Wrap a towel around the head

72. Using the theory of complimentary colors, what color of concealer will cover a bruise that is red?
    a. Beige
    b. White
    c. Green
    d. Brown

73. What kind of brush would be used to simulate pores in the skin?
    a. Tapered brush
    b. Flat tip brush
    c. Stipple brush
    d. Pointed brush

74. According to facial proportions, which of these equals the width of an eye?
    a. The width of the base of the nose
    b. One third the width of the mouth
    c. One fourth the width of the face
    d. One half the distance between the eyes

75. When a suture is used in an open wound or a similar area where there is a gap too large to be sutured together, a base must be provided for the wax that will fill that gap. It is provided using which of the following sutures?
    a. Purse string
    b. Worm
    c. Temporary
    d. Basket weave

76. When there is excessive swelling in the neck, a pattern of sutures can be made in the back of the neck. These points of entry and exit form which letter?
    a. V
    b. X
    c. M
    d. N

77. A gelatinous tissue filler is not the only substance that can be used hypodermically to rebuild tissue. Which of the following can also be used?
    a. Distilled water
    b. Lip wax
    c. Massage cream thinned with a little mineral oil
    d. Tissue filler solvent

78. If restoration attempts are unsuccessful or if damage is beyond restoration, which of the following is a good alternative for the family members?
    a. Allow them to see and hold an uninjured hand
    b. Show them any distinguishing tattoo(s)
    c. Show them an identifying mole or birthmark
    d. All of the above

79. Syphilis is contracted in the four ways identified below. Which one accounts for approximately 95 percent of cases?
    a. Sexual intercourse involving direct contact with fluids or lesions of an infected person
    b. Placental transmission
    c. Blood transfusion
    d. Kissing

80. The CDC lists at least nine hazardous body fluids. Which of the following is one of them?
    a. Urine
    b. Saliva
    c. Spinal fluid
    d. Perspiration

81. Which of the following is the agency that oversees procedures to prevent the spread of communicable diseases in the workplace?
    a. OSHA
    b. CDC
    c. NRA
    d. ADA

82. Which of the following types of hepatitis is classified as "highly contagious"?
    a. Hepatitis A
    b. Hepatitis B
    c. Hepatitis C
    d. Hepatitis D

83. Instruments that come into contact with HIV-contaminated blood should be cleaned with soap or detergent and water first, and then cleaned with a solution of 1:10 to 1:100 parts water (a quarter cup per gallon of water) and which of the following?
    a. Ammonia
    b. Bleach
    c. Milk
    d. Chlorine

84. Kaposi's sarcoma is sometimes seen in conjunction with which of the following?
    a. Gangrene
    b. Meningitis
    c. COPD
    d. AIDS

85. Healthy human cells are comprised of three parts: a nucleus, a cell (plasma) membrane, and:
    a. DNA
    b. RNA
    c. Cytoplasm
    d. Protoplasm

86. Acquired Immunodeficiency Syndrome (AIDS) can be transmitted through all of the following EXCEPT one. Which one is the exception?
    a. Saliva of an infected person
    b. Sexual contact
    c. Contact with contaminated blood
    d. Transplacental transmission from an infected mother

87. Which of the following is defined as an excess of fluid in interstitial spaces or cavities?
    a. Plasma
    b. Edema
    c. Hernia
    d. Sepsis

88. Influenza is a disease most known for attacking which system?
    a. Circulatory
    b. Respiratory
    c. Lymphatic
    d. Arterial

89. Current knowledge indicates that Creutzfeldt-Jakob disease is transmitted through which of the following?
    a. Sexual contact with an infected person
    b. Contact with the saliva of an infected person
    c. Airborne pathogens
    d. Contaminated corneal transplants

90. Which type of disease is the cause of more than half of the deaths in industrialized countries?
    a. Respiratory
    b. Lymphatic
    c. Cardiovascular
    d. Gastrointestinal

91. Lung infections that are prevalent among alcoholics and drug addicts are diseases of which system?
    a. Respiratory
    b. Cardiac
    c. Endocrine
    d. Nervous

92. Because of the chemical structure of embalming fluids, where is the best place to have an exhaust fan in the embalming room?
    a. Close to the embalming table near the floor
    b. In the ceiling
    c. High on the opposite wall near the ceiling
    d. Near the door

93. Gels used in the embalming process for an autopsied body have the same basic composition as which of the following types of chemicals?
    a. Jaundice fluids
    b. Cavity fluids
    c. Humectants
    d. Co-injection fluids

94. Fluids that work well with arterial embalming fluids but have a higher concentration of preservatives and disinfectants are called:
    a. Pre-injection fluids
    b. Co-injection fluids
    c. Cavity fluids
    d. Venous fluids

95. All of the following are types of arterial fluid preservatives EXCEPT:
    a. Aldehydes
    b. Phenolic compounds
    c. Formaldehyde "donor" compounds
    d. Humectants

96. Which of the following is the large opening at the base of the skull that is clearly exposed in a cranial autopsy?
    a. Circle of Willis
    b. Foramen magnum
    c. Diaphragm
    d. Interstitial space

97. The center of the circulatory system is the:
  a. Lungs
  b. Heart
  c. Arteries
  d. Veins

98. Where are the carotid artery and jugular vein located?
  a. Posterior to the sternocleidomastoid muscle
  b. Posterior to the trachea
  c. Posterior to the sternum
  d. Parallel to the ulnar artery

99. When embalming remains that have been autopsied, six arteries are usually used. Which of the following are two of them?
  a. Right and left femoral
  b. Right and left ulnar
  c. Right and left iliac
  d. Right and left jugular

100. There are three types of blood vessels: arteries, veins, and:
  a. Atria
  b. Ventricles
  c. Valves
  d. Capillaries

Answer Key

Arts

1. B: The deceased was of legal age. This requirement must be met for the will to take effect after the demise of the individual. A will completed by a minor who dies while still a minor is not recognized as a legal will. A codicil is a formal addition to a will, but it is not a requirement for a will to take effect. The legatee is the person who is to inherit the personal property specified in the will. Intestacy is the condition that occurs when a person dies and has no will.

2. C: The GPL for retention, and the casket and vault price list for reference only. The General Price List (GPL) is provided to the consumer for their retention. The funeral home cannot charge the consumer for a copy of the GPL. The casket and/or vault price list need to be handed to the consumer for reference as the products and prices are discussed, but the funeral director is not required by law to distribute them for retention. The Consumer Protection Fee applies to pre-need contracts. There is no requirement to compare prices requested by the consumer on dated company letterhead.

3. B: Constructive. Constructive custody in funeral service is the term applied to the custody rights that supersede actual custody rights, and they include the right of a party to control the disposition of the deceased. The person with actual custody may sometimes be a third party (such as a livery or public carrier), but someone else would maintain constructive custody at all times. Caveat emptor is Latin for "let the buyer beware." Consignment refers to merchandise shipped to an agent or to a customer. It does not take place as a result of an actual purchase, but under an agreement obliging the consignee to pay the consignor for the goods within a certain period of time once the merchandise is sold. Endowment refers to a permanent fund of property or money that is established to benefit an institution or person. An example is the sale of perpetual care cemetery property.

4. C: Funeral expenses, administration expenses, and taxes. In most states the funeral expenses of the deceased take top priority. This claim is immediately followed by the administration fees associated with settling the estate. Taxes come last. Taxes are not a preferred claim expense over the funeral expenses of the deceased in most states. Medical bills owed do not supersede taxes or funeral expenses in most states. Administration expenses are given less priority than funeral expenses and taxes in most states.

5. A: FTC. The Federal Trade Commission (FTC) is the government agency created to promote consumer protection and fair competition, and also to prevent anti-competitive commerce practices. The ICCFA is a national trade association for funeral homes and cemeteries, and serves as a resource for cemetery/funeral service professionals and the public. OSHA is the Occupational Safety Health Administration, and is a government agency created to prevent work-related injuries, illnesses, and fatalities by issuing and enforcing standards for workplace safety and health. The NFDA is the National Funeral Directors Association. It is not a government agency but a trade association for funeral directors. It serves as a resource for funeral service professionals and the public.

6. A: Tort. A tort occurs when a person takes a wrongful action against another person or property, and is a civil law matter. Mutilation as it relates to mortuary science is inflicting bodily damage or

injury on a person or animal by removing or destroying body parts. Obstruction occurs when a person or a situation creates an impasse or hinders someone from doing something. Replevin is an action to pick up goods or property by somebody who claims to own them and who promises to have the claim later tested in court. It does not apply to human remains.

7. B: Police power. Police power is based on constitutional law, and is the ability of the federal government and the states to order and be in command of certain prescribed legal actions necessary for the maintenance of public safety, health, order, and welfare. A tort is a wrongful action against a person or property, and is a civil law matter. A restrictive covenant is a deed restriction restraining the use of property in some prescribed manner. Uniform probate code is a statute passed by many states to varying degrees that spells out the laws that exist regarding the affairs of decedents and their estates.

8. B: Memorial service. A memorial service is always held without the casketed body. Funeral rite is a term that can describe both funerals and/or memorial services. Funeral, on the other hand, describes a service conducted when the body is present. During an entombment service, the human casketed body is placed in a crypt. A graveside service refers to one in which the deceased is in a casket. It is held at the cemetery interment site (grave) instead of a church or chapel. The casketed body is present at a traditional or complete cremation service, but at the end of the service the decreased goes to the crematory to be cremated instead of to the cemetery for interment burial.

9. C: VA form 90-2008. The APPLICATION FOR UNITED STATES FLAG FOR BURIAL PURPOSES, also known as VA form 90-2008, is the accepted document to apply for an American flag. The APPLICATION FOR BURIAL BENEFITS is the form to apply for burial benefits at the Veterans Administration. The STATEMENT OF DEATH BY FUNERAL DIRECTOR is a form completed by the funeral director to notify the Social Security Administration of the death. It is unrelated to the Veterans Administration. The APPLICATION FOR STANDARD GOVERNMENT HEADSTONE OR MARKER is for a memorial issued by the Veterans Administration.

10. A: Cot. The mortuary or ambulance cot is the most important item for transferring remains, and is a portable stretcher that has wheels, a mattress, and belts. It is used by both ambulances and funeral homes to move the injured and deceased. The flexible stretcher refers to the collapsible stretcher that folds so it can be carried up and down stairs. It can then be opened on site. The deceased can be placed on it and strapped in until they can be transferred to the cot. It is not the most important item for transfer since it is only used in special circumstances when access is difficult, such as in stairwells or elevators. The transfer vehicle refers to the actual motorized vehicle that transports the deceased from the place of death to the funeral home. The church truck is the portable device on wheels that can be extended to serve as a resting apparatus to display or move a casket in church or a funeral home.

11. A: i, ii, and iv. The purpose of the death certificate is to show vital statistics information and cause of death for medical or actuarial study, to serve as the legal permanent record of the deceased, and to serve as the legal record that final disposition has occurred. The Burial Cremation or Transit/Disposition Permit is a legal document issued by the proper government bureau authorizing transportation and/or disposition of human remains. It is the legal permit for the final disposition to take place.

12. A: Lead car, hearse, clergy, pallbearers, family cars/limo, and procession. Although some states may have requirements for processions to have a police car in the lead, the order of the cortege is typically: lead car, hearse, clergy, pallbearers, family cars/limo, and procession.

13. A: Narthex. The narthex is the entryway to the funeral home or church, and is also known as the lobby or foyer. The nave is the seating or audience section of the church. A niche is a permanent resting place for cremated remains typically found in a church or cemetery. A sanctuary is the area in the church where the public are seated during the service, and can also describe the area around the altar.

14. B: Sacrament of the Sick. The Sacrament of the Sick is an anointing ritual conducted by a priest. Catholics believe it is a rite in which God can help cure the critically ill or help prepare the souls of those who are dying for eternity. The Paschal candle is a large, white candle used in the Western rites of Christianity (Roman Catholic, Anglican, Lutheran, etc.). It is positioned near the casket during funeral masses. A Rosary Service is a sequence of Roman Catholic prayers. Rosary Beads, which consist of a string of beads and a crucifix, are used to count the prayers said during a Rosary Service.

15. C: Eucharist. The Eucharist is the name for the sanctified elements of Holy Communion, which comprise the essential rudiments for liturgical worship. The Paschal Candle is a large, white candle used in the Western rites of Christianity (Roman Catholic, Anglican, Lutheran, etc.) that is placed near the casket during funeral masses. The Communion Paten is a saucer-shaped plate usually made of precious metal that is held under the chin of the communicant to catch any particle of the Sacred Host that may fall. It is similar to the Mass Paten, but has a handle that projects outward. The Trisagion is the name for the three short blessings that are part of the funeral rites of the Eastern Orthodox faith.

16. D: Both B: and C:. The Declining Price Structure Model incorporates a lower margin on higher-priced caskets so the consumer CVI improves as they spend more. Both B: and C: are components of the Declining Price Structure Model. The Modified Declining Model places a lower margin on less expensive caskets.

17. C: Selected hardwood. Selected hardwood is a phrase used to describe a casket made of various trees, such as salix, poplar, or cottonwood. Single hinged panel refers to a casket lid that is in two sections. Wood veneer refers to the method of using glue during assembly to join a thin layer of superior wood to a layer of less costly wood so the superior wood is on top. A pine box is a casket made of wood from a pine tree.

18. B: Crushed. Casket interiors featuring a crushed style have a lining fabric placed on a metal form. Weights are added, and the material is then steamed and attached to an upholstery or backing. Masselin is the paper used in layers of sheets that is pressed and made up to provide an upholstery or backing. The extendover is the segment of the casket interior that extends over the top body molding. A tufted casket interior is made by inserting a padded material between a lining material and a backing material. Stitches are then added to create raised puffs.

19. A: Crepe. Crepe is a lightweight fabric lining cloth that has a slim, daintily crinkled or ridged facade made of silk, cotton, rayon, or wool. Satin is a fabric made of woven silk, nylon, or rayon that has a smooth, silky face. Velvet is a fabric made of woven silk, cotton, or rayon that has an evenly distributed, short, substantial, and dense pile. It is typically found in costlier caskets. Linen is a fabric made from the flax plant or non-flax fibers that are woven into a cross-section contour that contributes to the coarse consistency of the fabric.

20. A: Cenotaph. A cenotaph is a headstone or a commemorative plaque dedicated to deceased persons that are frequently interred in another location, such as the Vietnam War Memorial in Washington or at a cemetery's scattering garden for cremated remains. A crypt is a chamber in a mausoleum that is generally large enough to hold the casketed remains of one or several deceased persons. An epitaph is an inscribed message found on a monument describing the deeds or traits of the departed. A columbarium is a structure, room, or space in a mausoleum or other building that is a permanent resting place for cremated remains. It contains niches that are used to hold them.

21. D: Ferrous and non-ferrous. These are the two broad classifications of metal. Ferrous metals contain iron, and include steel and stainless steel. The other type of metal is non-ferrous. They are metals produced without iron or alloys that do not contain a considerable amount of iron, so they do not rust. Bronze is a non-ferrous metal alloy that must consist of at least 90 percent copper. Copper is a non-ferrous metallic element. Steel and stainless steel are ferrous metals formed from iron. Steel is a metal alloy made mostly of iron and carbon, and stainless steel is a metal alloy made of steel, chromium (at least 11 percent), and sometimes nickel. Galvanized steel is a ferrous metal coated with zinc.

22. D: Lug, arm, bar, and tip. The lug is the part of the handle that is connected to the body of the casket. The arm is the part of the handle that connects the bar to the lug. The bar is the part of the handle that attaches to the lug or arm. It is what the pallbearers hold while moving the casket. The tip is the decorative piece attached to the last part of the bar. The rim is the molding in the casket cap. The shell is the body and the lid of the casket.

23. D: Stainless steel. Stainless steel is a metal alloy made of steel, chromium (at least 11 percent), and sometimes nickel. Copper is a non-ferrous metallic element; it is not an alloy. Non-ferrous metal is any metal formed without iron. Bronze is a non-ferrous metal alloy. It must consist of at least 90 percent copper, and is measured in ounces per square foot. Steel is a metal alloy made mostly of iron and carbon.

24. C: Attending. Attending is when the listener, in this case the funeral director, listens with unbroken interest and observes the speaker for non-verbal body language while maintaining eye contact. Adaptive refers to a form of modern funeral rite that is flexible and can be changed in any way those who are involved see fit. Paraphrasing is a listening skill in which the listener, in this case the funeral director, restates the core communication the family provided so he/she can verify what was said and that the message was understood correctly. Summarizing refers to the communication by the funeral director at the end of the conference. It is when detailed choices such as merchandise selections and the key points of the tangible contract agreement are assessed in front of the purchaser so the ultimate agreement can be verified.

25. D: Denial, anger, bargaining, depression, and acceptance. Denial, anger, bargaining, depression, and acceptance are the five stages of dying identified by Dr. Elisabeth Kubler-Ross in her book On Death and Dying. Accept, express, adjust, and reinvest refer to the Tasks of Mourning outlined by J. William Worden. In this theory, he describes the route whereby the person accepts the reality of the loss and experiences the expressive pain, then adjusts to the condition where the deceased is not there, and finally re-invests into another relationship. Numbness, yearning, disorganization and despair, and reorganization refer to the four phases of mourning described by Bowlby. Shock, awareness of loss, conservation-withdrawal, healing, and renewal refer to the phases of the mourning process as described by Sanders.

26. B: Bereavement. Bereavement is the experience a person goes through subsequent to a loss when they are grieving and mourning the loss of a loved one. Mourning is the process one goes through after the loss of someone as they reorganize their life without the person. Thanatology is the study of dying, death, and grief. Grief is the emotional reaction that results from the loss of a loved one.

27. A: Grief syndrome. Grief syndrome is the term used to describe the most common and ordinary patterns and assortment of feelings and behaviors people exhibit following the loss of a loved one. Guilt is blaming oneself for something that has occurred. Shame is the assumption of blame aimed at oneself in the presence of others. Attachment theory is John Bowlby's concept that for safety and security reasons, people develop long-lasting attachments to specific persons when they are very young.

28. C: Anger. Anger is an expression of aggravation and helplessness, and it is important for funeral directors to comprehend that this emotion may be directed at them by grieving clients. Guilt is blaming oneself for something that has happened. Caused by a loss, grief is an emotion or set of emotions heightened during mourning. Mourning is an adjustment process that involves grief or sorrow experienced over a period of time.

29. C: Chronic grief. Chronic grief is excessive, and continues for an extended period of time. The individual is aware that it doesn't seem to be coming to a finish. Masked grief is when a person is oblivious to the fact that their symptoms (physical and behavioral) are related to a loss. The person does not permit oneself to express grief. Delayed grief is when a person deliberately postpones or suppresses the natural grief reaction. Exaggerated grief is an escalation of a normal grief reaction. It can result in various medical conditions, including clinical depression or anxiety disorder.

30. C: Grief counseling. Grief counseling involves communicating with those who have lost a loved one recently and are mourning to facilitate the bereavement process and help them move through the stages of grief. At-need counseling is providing informational services to families subsequent to the death of a person. An example is when a funeral director provides a GPL to quote prices on various service selections. Grief therapy is typically one-on-one counseling for those who are unable to move through and complete the stages of mourning. Typically, the person in need of this type of therapy is having a delayed grief reaction or an exaggerated grief response, or is demonstrating physical or behavioral symptoms that remain unresolved.

31. B: Samuel Rogers. In 1868, Samuel Rogers patented the trocar, which is used to inject and drain excess fluids. The English doctor Dr. William Harvey (1578-1657) is credited with the discovery and documentation of the circulation of the frog. Gabriel Clauderus is the German individual who is credited with developing the practice of injecting lye into the veins to embalm a deceased individual. The formerly accepted practice was evisceration. James A. Gray is the individual who received the first patent for a metallic coffin.

32. D: The sun and the cult of Osiris. The sun and the cult of Osiris refer to the god of the Underworld and the judge of the dead in Egyptian culture, respectively. A Pagan is one who is not extremely religious or is not religious at all. Pagans do not identify with the God of the Bible, or with the teachings of the Torah or the Koran. Natron is a sodium carbonate mineral (salt) that was a key embalming element used by the Egyptians. Canopic jars were the four jars used in Egyptian culture that contained a portion of the viscera of the deceased. The tops had an image representing each of the four sons of Horus. Horus was the son of Isis and Osiris. The Kher-heb was the Egyptian priest who was the embalming practitioner and also had the responsibility of making funeral

arrangements with the family. The Libitinarius was the Roman head undertaker who made funeral arrangements with the family in Roman times.

33. D: Wool. The Burial in Woolen Act of 1666 required the use of woolen cloth instead of linen for the inside layer of the coffin. The purpose was to support goods manufactured in England, and there was a monetary penalty for disobedience. Velvet refers to a fabric made of woven silk, cotton, or rayon that has a consistently dispersed, short, thick, dense pile. It is usually found in costlier caskets. Masselin is the hard-pressed paper used in layers of sheets that serve as an upholstery or backing. Satin is a fabric made of woven silk, nylon, or rayon that has a smooth and silky face.

34. A: Nuclear family. A nuclear family is a household that includes one man, one woman, and their children. An extended (joint) family includes the father and mother and all of their children (except married daughters), as well as their son's wives and their children (except married daughters). A daughter becomes part of her husband's family when she gets married. The modified extended family is a type of nuclear family in which one nuclear family is connected to another because the two are related by marriage or are close friends. This characteristic is important since more than one household is required to have a modified extended family and these households include at least one additional man and/or one additional woman. The blended family consists of one male and one female and their children from previous marriages, as well as any children they may have together.

35. C: Nuclear family. A nuclear family is a household that includes one man, one woman, and their children. This type of family has characteristics likely to make them more open to a contemporary funeral rite. These characteristics include the fact that nuclear families may exhibit class and geographic mobility. They may also be matriarchal, patriarchal, or egalitarian since both husband and wife typically work. An extended (joint) family includes the father and mother and all of their children (except married daughters), as well as their son's wives and their children (except married daughters). This type of arrangement is typical of the Amish and Native Americans, groups not likely to be open to contemporary funeral rites or cremation. The bureaucratization family is not a classification of a family structure, but is a concept in sociology that refers to the management of an organization that has many controls and adheres to rules and regulations. These attributes are typical of governments in urban areas. The demographic family is a grouping or a market segment of a certain demographic.

36. D: Sociology. Sociology is the science that studies various social groups and how individuals behave and relate to each other as a group in relation to other social groups. This can influence funeral service disposition arrangements. Funeralization is the practice of the funeral itself, including a variety of activities linked to the final disposition. This includes the type of service and the merchandise needed to accommodate the funeral service. Ethnocentrism is the belief that one's ethnic or cultural group, nation, race, or culture is better than all other groups. Pathology is the science that studies the origin, nature, and track of diseases.

37. D: Neo-localism. Neo-localism refers to an inclination in society for people to move away from where they were born and raised and relocate to a new region for vocation or weather. Enculturation refers to the process by which certain values and customs become more embedded in our behaviors as we grow up. As it relates to funeral arrangements, a person making funeral arrangements for a deceased relative who was raised in a certain social class may have pre-conceived ideas of how a funeral service should be performed (such as in a church or chapel) and the goods and services that should be part of the funeral service. Ethnocentrism is the belief that one's ethnic or cultural group, nation, race, or culture is superior to all other groups. Social

stratification is the categorizing of people according to their financial status or worth, as well as their social status in the community.

38. D: Assignee. When an assignment is made, a party transfers legal rights to another person who is called an assignee. The assignor is the party who is making the assignment. A beneficiary is the person who will receive a stated gain of some kind, such as the life insurance proceeds pursuant to a life insurance policy, or the person who will inherit property, such as that declared in a will. A consignee is the individual to whom goods are shipped, usually via a common carrier.

39. B: Bailment. Bailment is the provisional transfer of custody but not the permanent transfer of title of personal possessions between two persons. A consignee is the individual to whom goods are shipped, usually via a common carrier. A blank endorsement is an endorsement on a bill of exchange that does not recognize a specific payee, and so it may compensate the bearer. Acceptance occurs when parties agree on an offer, which in turn results in a tangible contract.

40. A: Maker. The maker is the entity or individual who makes the guarantee to pay, and is the signer of the promissory note. The payee is the entity or individual to whom the pledge of monies is made. The drawee is the entity or individual selected and required to make the payment of finances. It is from their monies the draft is drawn. The drawer is an entity or person that draws or executes an order for the disbursement of money.

41. A: Statement of operations. The statement of operations, also called the income statement, is a written report that identifies the financial profitability of a company over a precise period of time. The balance sheet is a written report that shows recorded assets, liabilities, and owners' equity of the company in fiscal terms. A statement of financial position is another name for the balance sheet, and it contains the same information as the balance sheet. A trial balance is a register of all the general ledger accounts. The accounts' respective debit or credit balances are itemized in the business's ledger.

42. B: Working capital. Working capital is the tangible working liquidity that is accessible for use by a company. The statement of operations, also called the income statement, is a written statement that identifies the financial profitability of a company over a precise period of time. Proving cash is when a business authenticates that the cash it has on hand and in the bank is equal to the amount listed in the accounting documentation. Useful life is the number of years that a business asset or piece of property can be depreciated, and is established by the IRS.

43. D: The Federal Insurance Contributions Act. The Federal Insurance Contributions Act (FICA) is a compulsory United States payroll taxation that the federal government collects to fund social security. Federal Income Tax Withholding is the federally mandated law that requires salaries and wages to be subject to having taxes withheld. The Federal Unemployment Tax Act (FUTA) refers to the payroll taxation imposed by the federal government that is used to compensate individuals who qualify if they become unemployed. A W-2 is a wage and tax statement generated by the employer and given to each eligible employee to delineate earnings, deductions, and taxes for the previous full year of employment.

44. C: Note receivable. A note receivable is a written agreement of obligation by a customer to repay a defined debt to a business. It also outlines the agreed-upon terms of repayment. Federal Income Tax Withholding is the federally mandated law that requires salaries and wages to be subject to having taxes withheld. A maker is the entity or individual who makes the guarantee to pay, and is

the signer of the promissory note. A blank endorsement is an endorsement on a bill of exchange that does not recognize a specific payee, and so it may compensate the bearer.

45. D: Both B: and C:. A compact disc and a jump drive are alternative storage devices for recorded digital data. The stored data can be viewed by connecting to certain electronic equipment. A scanner is a peripheral device that records a document and/or image in a digital format, and allows for the image to be replicated.

46. C: Needs and wants, software and hardware. Determining the purposes a computer will be used for is the foremost consideration when deciding which computer system to purchase. The software programs designed to carry out a particular task are important to complete specific assignments, and the hardware is important to meet the processing needs of the software. Viruses and spam are items that relate to Internet security protection, and are not the first points of consideration when purchasing a computer system. Microsoft and Apple are two of the leading computer manufacturers, and both are relatively satisfactory in terms of their capabilities. Wi-Fi, or Wireless Fidelity, is a technology that makes the mobile use of laptop computers and other devices possible, and is not the most critical component of making a computer purchasing decision. The Internet is a global system of interconnected computer networks, and it is not the most critical component of a computer purchasing decision.

47. C: Frederick Herzberg. Frederick Herzberg was the psychologist who authored "The Two Factor Theory" and proposed the concept that peoples' motivation in the workplace is influenced by multiple factors that lead to an overall feeling of satisfaction or dissatisfaction. Abraham Maslow did not write "The Two Factor Theory," but he did author several psychology papers regarding motivation. These theorized that people have a hierarchical ladder of simple to complex needs that they strive to achieve. Douglas McGregor was a teacher who developed a management theory in which he classified peoples' work behavior and motivation as fitting into two groups. He categorized workers as Theory X or Theory Y, and suggested that creating an environment for each type of worker could contribute to their motivation.

48. D: Equal Employment Opportunity Act. The Equal Employment Opportunity Act of 1972 was enacted to make any employment discrimination illegal. This included denying a candidate on the basis of race, religion, color, national origin, and sex. It was developed to ensure applications from all qualified candidates would be evaluated fairly by the potential employer. OSHA is the Occupational Safety Health Administration and the creator of the Occupational Safety and Health Act. Its role as a government body is to avoid work-related injuries, illnesses, and fatalities by developing written standards for workplace safety and health, making them available to employers, and enforcing penalties for non-compliance. The Immigration Reform and Control Act is national legislation that requires an employer to check and authenticate that job applicants are legally sanctioned to work in the United States, either because they are citizens or because they are approved aliens. The Age Discrimination Employment Act states that employer decisions regarding hiring, layoffs, merit increases, etc. can be classified as discriminatory and illegal if it is found that they were made on the basis that an employee was over the age of 40.

49. D: Stare Decisis. Stare Decisis is the theory of law that purports that an established past court decision can be a model to provide insight for a future case since the court is likely to uphold the basis of law used to make the previous conclusion. Statute of Limitations is a law that creates a set time limit to pursue legal action and certain forms of litigation after the action in question occurred. Statutes are legal policies formed by legislation that direct the administration of acceptable behaviors in a state, city, or country. The Equal Employment Opportunity Act of 1972 was enacted

to make any employment discrimination illegal. This included denying a candidate on the basis of race, religion, color, national origin, and sex. It was developed to ensure applications from all qualified candidates would be evaluated fairly by the potential employer.

50. B: Debt equity. Debt equity is a gauge that represents a business's financial leverage, is determined by dividing the business's total liabilities by stockholders' equity, and also represents how much funding has been borrowed to finance the business. The current ratio is the mathematical proportion that quantifies the capability of a company to pay short-term debt commitments. It is calculated by taking the current assets and dividing their value by the current liabilities. The book value is the reported economic worth of an asset as it is cataloged on the balance sheet of the business documentation. Economic order quantity is the ideal quantity of inventory a business should keep in stock to curtail the total inventory asset expenses and ordering overhead.

51. C: Physiological factors are the third influence. Internal factors are psychological and external are sociological. Although illogical behavior may be displayed during grief, it is not one of the three main factors.

52. C: Most Native American tribes do believe in an afterlife but there are exceptions, such as the Navajo tribe. Most tribes believe that birth and death are equally sacred. Although some do believe the body is a shell, others do not. They talk to it and visit it.

53. A: Death defiance is when people defy death, thinking they can take things with them and that death does not deprive them of anything.

54. D: Preparation of the body of a deceased Jew is called tahara, and is done by the chevra kadisha, or holy society. Shiva is the period of mourning after the death and Yahrzeit is the first anniversary of the death.

55. A: Suicide is the other form of violent death. It is essentially homicide at one's own hand.

56. D: All of the situations are ones that most people would not share with others. The bereaved would therefore experience complicated grief when the death occurs.

57. C: Tradition is also a big influence on a person's perspective. Gender, race, and financial status may be factors in other facets of life, but ideas about death are more influenced by religion, family, culture, and observed and experienced traditions.

58. B: Although all of the choices are types of nonverbal communication, paralanguage is the one in which a person's words do not match the tone of their speech.

59. A: Aftercare is the practice of helping families in various ways after the services are over. Preneed is helping people plan for services before they need them, and the arrangement conference is the meeting with families to plan services before they occur. Complicated grief is a type of grief.

60. D: Allowing them to bring in personal items will help them in their grief. It will be helpful not only to have them at the services, but also to gather them at home. All of the other choices are sometimes thought to be offers of assistance to make things easier, but they don't help the family deal with their grief.

61. A: They do not always occur in the order in which they're usually listed. Because everyone is different, so is their grief. They take different amounts of time to get through not only the stages, but grief itself. Making a deal with God is called "bargaining."

62. C: Adults should let children participate in funerals if a child expresses a desire to do so. A child should also be told of the death as soon after the death as possible, be encouraged to go to the cemetery, and be encouraged to talk to other people about it.

63. B: All of them are significant but people tend to recognize the grief of all family members except those who experience the death of a sibling. It is a specific and unique grief, and needs to be acknowledged.

64. D. Each must be notified when planning the type of service described in the question.

65. A: The cloth covering that is placed on the casket in a Catholic church is called a pall. If a flag is on the casket going into the church, it must be removed before the pall can be placed on the casket. A flag cannot be placed under or over the pall.

66. B: A clergy person is always going to appreciate not only your honesty but your willingness to learn how he/she wants things to be done for the service.

67. B: All the other choices meet the requirement of having the body in a rigid container. Just imagine the awkwardness involved in getting a body into the retort wrapped in a sheet, with nothing sturdy underneath it to get it in safely.

68. D: A veteran with a discharge other than "dishonorable" is entitled to military honors. This means one with an "honorable" or "general" discharge is eligible. Rank is inconsequential, as is whether death occurred during wartime.

69. B: Although all of them are components of the arrangement conference, the most important one is listening. A funeral director can't make arrangements for services that will meet or even exceed the customer's expectations unless he or she practices careful listening.

70. D: Green cemetery guidelines do not permit an embalmed body to be buried there, as those who develop these rules believe that the embalming chemicals contaminate the ground and affect public systems. They typically do allow the body to be dressed and also placed in a casket, but dictate that the clothing and casket must be made of natural fibers and materials.

71. D: To ship remains, they must be sent with a burial/transmit permit.

72. C: A family member can provide a container for a person's cremated remains. A cemetery may have regulations for an urn vault if it will be buried, but there is no mention of a cemetery burial in the question.

73. A: A bailee is a person who accepts property. Despite the similarity of the term to the word "bail," it is not related to crime. A mediator is one who works to achieve an agreement between two parties. A conservator is a person appointed to care for another person, and a codicil is an addendum to a will.

74. A: Libel is a picture or written statement that can damage a person's reputation. Immunity gives a person freedom from a penalty in exchange for something. Grand larceny is theft of an item higher in value than one that would result in a charge of petty larceny. Habeas corpus is bringing a prisoner before the court to decide if detention is warranted.

75. C: A fiduciary is a person or institution who keeps money for someone else. An assignee is someone who assigns goods to another person, a devisee is a person designated in a will to receive property, and a distributee is one who receives property from the deceased's personal representative.

76. B: An agreement to provide something for something is quid pro quo. In this question, the funeral director agrees to provide services and merchandise and the purchaser agrees to pay an agreed upon sum of money.

77. A: When a person gives someone else the right to claim something that belongs to her, it is known as an assignment. She is assigning it, or signing it over, to someone else.

78. B: A confidentiality agreement makes the prospective purchaser promise to keep all information discussed, financial and otherwise, confidential.

79. D: Obviously, if there are other embalmers who are in the room doing other work, it's allowed. Most states have laws that allow a medical doctor to observe the embalming process and even a member of the deceased's family. Any non-licensed people are prohibited, even if it's the embalmer's husband or wife.

80. C: A legal divorce severs the relationship that once made the former spouse the next-of-kin. A medical doctor may have many rights, but signing a cremation authorization is not one of them, unless he/she is the deceased's legal next-of-kin. The same thing applies to a member of the clergy. Many states now recognize an agent assignment made by the deceased during his life that gives the agent specific powers. The assignment must specify the right to authorize cremation in writing.

81. D: The Federal Trade Commission's Funeral Rule requires that the funeral director provide the General Price List as soon as any mention of prices or costs is brought up. It doesn't matter if the customer asks about this as soon as they sit down or if it's out of the order that the funeral director follows when meeting with a family. It must be provided as soon as the consumer asks questions about costs.

82. C: 60 percent of 9 is 5.4, which means that five are not enough, but six are because at 66.6 percent it is more than 60 percent.

83. D: The FTC Funeral Rule does not require you to send a copy of your General Price List to a caller; however, sending one may show the caller how helpful you are. You are required, though, to answer their pricing questions using the costs listed on your GPL. Individuals do not have to come into your funeral home to get prices.

84. D: If a family asks for the body to be embalmed, you must do it. If they choose services such as direct burial or direct cremation, embalming is not necessary. The FTC Funeral Rule does not require embalming. Remains do not have to be embalmed to be shipped out of town because religious or other customs may allow the deceased to be shipped using dry ice or other means.

85. A: The funds can be deposited into a state funeral directors' association's trust fund, an account at a local bank, or, in some states, in an insurance policy or annuity. Under no circumstances is it legal for the entire amount to be deposited into a funeral home's bank account.

86. B: If a person on Medicaid dies and has a burial account, the funds must be paid to the Medicaid office. Before all of a person's assets and funds are exhausted through paying the costs of their own nursing home or other care, they are permitted to set aside funds to pay for their own funeral expenses. Medicaid then takes over the financial responsibility of paying the high cost of their care. It's only fair, then, that the amount not used for its intended purpose be returned to the agency that has paid thousands of dollars for care. The other choices are prohibited by law.

87. D: It is against the law to display any casket without a price on it. There are no laws that prohibit grouping caskets by type or price, or from showing pictures in lieu of actual caskets.

88. C: Using a computer that has photos of caskets is another way to show them to consumers. The lists given as choices are exactly what the name says: lists. They do not show photos, just prices and descriptions.

89. B: Although many funeral homes display full-size vaults, cross sections of vaults, or vault photos, the most important part of displaying burial vaults is being able to provide a knowledgeable, accurate description to the consumer of each, including their advantages.

90. A: All the other choices involve the funeral director taking some action to facilitate a decision by the customer. Having products or photos of products around is a subtle way of showing them. The customer is allowed to initiate conversation about the items and possibly decide to purchase them.

91. A: Prayer cards and memorial folders can easily be created and printed on a computer. Surprisingly, there are still many funeral homes that don't give families the option to choose prayers or add a photo.

92. B: An informational brochure is a great promotional tool that can be displayed at the arrangement conference and in a visible place during services. It should describe why your funeral home is exceptional. A General Price List is not a merchandising piece. It is informational only. Urn displays and pictures of monuments are used to promote objects, not services.

93. D: Email is sent from a different type of program. Registration cards can be printed from a computer, but not by using the funeral home software. Although most providers of funeral home software will also help you design and publish a website, it is not done with the funeral home software program.

94. B: An accounting program is designed to do calculations and organize numerical data. It can do this faster than a calculator and with fewer keystrokes. Email might help you stay in touch with people, but it won't organize or calculate numerical information.

95. C: Payroll is a liability; the other choices are assets.

96. B: Depreciation can be claimed on tangible assets that will decrease in value. The only choice given that is an asset is vehicles.

97. B: Amounts owed for funeral services are included in accounts receivable. Therefore, the amount in accounts receivable will decrease when an amount that is owed is paid.

98. B: A website will provide lots of helpful information to your customers. This may include obituaries, prices, grief resources, facts about your funeral home, and other helpful information. You can post pictures of your children, but that's less important than providing consumer information. A website will not help with your accounting needs, and although you can send email through some websites, this feature is not as important as the information you're providing on the website pages.

99. A: A scanner will scan a picture and load it onto your computer. From there, it can then be inserted into the cards or folders. Although you could use a digital camera to take a picture of the picture, it would then have to be uploaded to the computer, and would therefore be a second generation photo. This photo would be of lower quality than a scanned one.
100. C: A trial balance will show the profits and losses of a business. It will not track inventory, help with vehicle maintenance, or ensure accurate payroll.

Science

1. C: High index fluids. High index fluids are for situations in which the preservation demand is high due to the condition of the deceased. These chemicals usually have an index higher than 30. The harsher the conditions of the body, the stronger the primary solution should be. Low index fluids typically have a formaldehyde index in the range of 10 to 18, and it is not advisable to use them in high demand preservation circumstances. The use of these fluids results in the tissue remaining moist and natural with a soft to medium-firm texture. It is not wise to use them in situations where there is high water retention. Humectants are chemicals that increase the tissues' ability to maintain moisture, and aid in preventing dehydration. It would not be advisable to use them in situations where there is already too much moisture, as this would only further inhibit preservation. Water conditioning is an additive agent to remove or render ineffective various chemicals in water that may inhibit drainage or preservation. It does not specifically address the needs that are present in high-demand preservation situations.

2. A: After embalming. Tissue builder doesn't contain embalming fluid so it must be used after a corpse has been embalmed to shape treated tissue. If it was used before embalming, the subsequent embalming treatment would not be capable of effectively reaching the tissue that had not been preserved.

3. D: The embalming case report. The embalming case report is the all-encompassing written record that includes a drawn sketch diagramming the condition of the body. It identifies the deceased and the embalming practitioner, as well as the chemicals used, the time elapsed, and the funeral home procedures performed. Putrefaction is a term used to describe the decomposition of proteins by diverse enzymes as well as the actions of anaerobic bacteria. It is not the title of a case report. Decomposition is the breakdown of compounds into simpler substances by microbes and autolytic enzymes. The level of decomposition is one finding listed in the embalming case report. Sanitation refers to the documentable efforts to provide for personal and environmental hygiene while working around a corpse. The body and its immediate environment are unsanitary, and create a hazardous condition that could result in an infection to the embalming practitioner.

Sanitation is not addressed in a separate report, but the use of chemicals should be listed in the embalming case report so that there is a record of sanitization efforts.

4. D: Both A: and B:. Licensees and those authorized by the family or the state. Any person who has a license to perform work in the preparation room in accordance with the rules and regulations of the state in which they are practicing and the authorization of the business is allowed to be in the prep room. Additionally, any approved family member or state authorized personnel is permitted to be in the prep room. Pre-need counselors typically have no authorization to enter the prep room. They are business agents authorized to represent cemetery and/or funeral products and services to clients in advance of a death.

5. D: Both b and c, differential pressure and rate of flow. Differential pressure is the difference between the potential pressure reading and the actual pressure reading. It is a gauge of the rate of flow, which is the amount of embalming solution that enters the body in a given period. A vacuum breaker is an accessory device that prevents water from flowing backwards into an unintended water source, which would result in contamination or pollution.

6. C: Aneurism needle. An aneurism needle is a small, razor-sharp medical apparatus used in embalming. It is commonly used to make incisions into tissues, including the initial incision in the corpse for the "raising" of the carotid artery and jugular vein for injection and drainage. A bistoury knife is a long, pointed medical utensil commonly used for removing excess body tissues. A hemostat (forceps) is used to compress blood vessels and limit or prevent blood flow passage or drainage.

7. D: Thanatology. Thanatology is the analysis and study of death and dying and the states of affairs that are pressing on those involved. It evaluates how various factors integrate to influence a person's behavior. Psychology is the analysis and study of human and animal behavior and rationale, including how unique environmental circumstances influence behavior. Psychiatry is the scientific study of both mental and emotional abnormalities in people in order to provide treatment management options. Psychiatry patients include persons affected by a death. Pathology is the scientific examination of diseases in animals, including how the disease was contracted as well as how it affects the physical well-being of the animal.

8. A: Agonal hypostasis. Agonal hypostasis is a symptomatic progression by which blood pools and settles in the lowest parts of the body as a result of gravity. Hemolysis occurs when the walls of red blood cells are broken down and the hemoglobin they contain is released. Intermittent drainage (restricted drainage) is a method of drainage used during embalming that stops and starts the drainage at intervals while embalming fluid is being injected. Agonal mortis is the condition that occurs after a person is deceased. There is a progression of temperature reduction as the body temperature of the corpse decreases.

9. B: Hydrolysis. Hydrolysis in a corpse is a chemical change in which the water in the cadaver splits apart the cells' chemical bonds as the body decomposes. This process is the fundamental accelerator of decomposition. Hemolysis is the process by which red blood cells break down and the hemoglobin they contain is released because it is no longer confined by the cell walls. Hematemesis is the state or condition of a person who is in the act of vomiting blood. Fermentation is a chemical process during which a fluid or solid goes through a chemical change over a period of time and the result is the release of energy.

10. D: All of the above. Rigor mortis can be broken down by the use of physical methods, including flexing, bending, rotating, and massaging the affected joints.

11. D: Both B: and C:. The Centers for Disease Control (CDC) has determined through studies conducted with practicing funeral directors that the most common bloodborne and airborne pathogens contracted through exposure to dead human bodies are staphylococcal infections and cutaneous (skin) tuberculosis. A staphylococcal infection is a very contagious malady that can be transmitted from person to person from droplets from the nose of an infected person or from the bacteria in the pus oozing out of an infected lesion. Cutaneous tuberculosis (TB) is tuberculosis on the skin caused by the mycobacterium tuberculosis, and if the embalmer is exposed to this a skin infection called tuberculosis chancre may occur. A hematoma is due to a leaking blood vessel, and results in an area with a collected pool of blood.

12. D: 12 – 20. Air exchanges per hour refers to the movement of a volume of air in a given period of time. According to the Mortuary College textbook Embalming: History, Theory & Practice by Robert Mayer, the exchange rate should be between 12 and 20 exchanges per hour for ventilation to be considered adequate. Air exchange rates of between 5 – 8 or 5–10 exchanges per hour are not adequate. Air exchange rates of 20 – 30 per hour are higher than necessary.

13. C: Centrifugal pump. The centrifugal pump is a relatively contemporary device compared to all the other choices because it uses an electric pump to produce pressure that can be delivered with or without a pulsating effect. The bulb syringe was a device that was used in the past in embalming. It was manually squeezed to deliver and release pressure and the ensuing flow. The gravity bottle was a frequently used historic technique of embalming that used the force of gravity to move embalming fluids. The hand pump was another device historically used for embalming that relied on the manual action of one's hand to create pressure and move fluid.

14. D: Ventral. Ventral is an anatomical expression used to refer to the anterior or frontal portion of the human body. Dorsal is an anatomical phrase used to describe the posterior or rear of the human body. Anatomical position is the recognized scientific standard of how a human body should be situated so that all directions and positions are determined in the same way. Medial refers to the midline area (medial plane) of the human body.

15. B: Intradermal suture. The intradermal suture (hidden suture) is used to secure incisions so the ligature remains concealed under the skin. The basket weave suture (cross stitch) is a system of stitches that crosses the limits of an excision to secure fillers and hold tissues in their proper positions. The bridge stitch (interrupted suture) is a short-term suture made up of divided pieces that are tied to hold the tissue in its proper position. They are removed later. The loop stitch is a single stitch used to secure restorative materials.

16. D: Angulus oris eminence. The angulus oris eminence is a natural face marking that consists of a comparatively undersized, convex, raised area found lateral to the end of the line of closure of the mouth. The angulus oris sulcus is a natural facial marking groove found at each end of the line of closure of the mouth. The frontal process of the maxilla is the raised part of the upper jaw that protrudes slightly as it rises alongside the nasal bone to meet the frontal bone in the upper jaw. The frontal eminences are a pair of distinctive raised areas of the frontal bone found roughly one inch beneath the normal hairline.

17. A: Approximately three to six hours after embalming. Most funeral homes will allow several hours to pass after embalming before applying mortuary wax so the tissue is treated and becomes

firm and dry. Restorative wax is typically applied to replace skin and make a "skin-like surface" from an area of fever blisters, abrasions, or burns. Surface wax needs to be applied to embalmed tissue. At least three hours of setting time is required following embalming for the embalming treatment to infiltrate and dry all tissues. The application of surface wax to tissue immediately after embalming is not recommended since the surface areas of the deceased at this point are not preserved or firm. It is not necessary to wait 24 hours for the tissues to reach a sufficient state of preservation before applying mortuary wax.

18. B: Convex profile. The convex profile is the most common profile form among human beings. In this form, a person's forehead posteriorly recedes from the eyebrows and the chin recedes from the upper lip. A vertically balanced profile is when the chin, forehead, and upper lip are all situated in a related alignment so none of them protrude or recede more than the other two features. A concave profile is when the forehead of the person protrudes further than the eyebrows and the chin protrudes beyond the plane of the upper lip. There is no such thing as a horizontal balanced profile.

19. D: Closed or greenstick fracture. A greenstick fracture is a bowed or unfinished fracture (closed fracture) because the broken bone does not perforate the skin and there is no exposed bone. A compound fracture is a type of fracture in which the wound causes the broken bone to slice and push through the skin. Third degree is not a fracture classification, but is used to classify burns when the victim's skin tissues have been charred. An open fracture is the same as a compound fracture. In this type of fracture, an injury causes a broken bone to pierce through the skin.

20. B: Purse suture. A purse suture is a stitch that is used to close a rounded opening. It is made by stitching around the perimeter and pulling the stitches firmly to close the borders of the opening. The basket weave suture (cross stitch) is a system of stitches that traverses the boundaries of an incision and is used to secure fillers and keep body tissues in place. The bridge suture (interrupted suture) is a transitory suture consisting of independently cut and tied stitches that is used to maintain the location of tissues. The whip suture is used to secure elongated incisions, such as those made during an autopsy.

21. C: Opaque. Opaque cosmetics are used to cover something like a blemish or discoloration from view since they do not permit light to pass through them. Translucent cosmetics are used to diminish the appearance of something but not hide it from view since they allow diffused light to pass through. A transparent cosmetic is one that is used when there is no need to hide any blemish or discoloration. An aerosol is a medium for spraying a product that uses a gas propellant. In the case of cosmetics, an aerosol can spray ones that are opaque, translucent, or transparent.

22. B: Oval. The oval head shape is the most common head shape. When viewed from the front, the cheekbones are wider than the cranium and the cranium is a little bit wider than the lower jaw. The diamond head shape is the widest when viewed from the front. It is also characterized by wide cheekbones and a narrow forehead and jaw line. The round head shape is short and features full cheeks, a full jaw line, and a rounded cranium. The oblong head shape is long and narrow. The forehead and the chin may be rounded or square.

23. D: Angulus oris sulcus. The angulus oris sulcus is a natural facial marking groove found at each end of the line of closure of the mouth. The weather line is the line of color change at the junction of the wet and dry portions of the upper and lower segment of each mucous membrane. The medial lobe is the tiny raised portion on the midline of the upper mucous membrane. The angulus oris eminence is a natural facial marking that is a raised, convex contour lateral to the end of the line of closure of the mouth.

24. A: Parietal. The parietal bones are the two area bones of the cranium as well as the apex piece of the cranium. The occipital bones are situated in the lower back region of the cranium. The temporal bone includes the lowermost sides and base of the cranium. The zygomatic bones are the diamond-shaped bones that outline the cheekbones.

25. B: Temporalis. Temporalis is the name of one of the facial muscles. It is the strongest chewing muscle, and aids in the side-to-side and up-and-down movement of the mandible. The temporal is a bone, not a muscle, of the cranium. The levator labii superioris is the muscle that moves and lifts the upper lip. The corrugators are muscles that move the eyebrow inferiorly and medially. They can also form a frown when they are tightened.

26. D: Nasolabial sulcus. The nasolabial sulcus is a furrow that is not present at birth. It starts at the superior border of the wing of the nose and extends to the side of the mouth. As one gets older, it gets more noticeable. The nasal sulcus is a natural facial marking present at birth that is found between the posterior margins of the wing of the nose and the nasolabial fold. The nasolabial fold is a natural facial marking present at birth. It is found on the cheek bordering the corners of the mouth. The philtrum is a natural facial marking present at birth. It is a vertical line found medially on the upper lip that is sandwiched between the columnar nasi and the medial lobe on the mucous membrane of the upper lip.

27. D: Bacillus. Bacillus bacteria are typically shaped like cylindrical rods. Bacillus is one of the three general groups of bacteria categorized based on their cellular shape. Vibrio bacteria have a curved shape. Vibrio is a sub-classification of the spiral-shaped group, which is one of the three general groups of bacteria cellular shapes. Coccus bacteria typically have a spherical shape, and make up one of the three general groups of bacteria categorized by their cellular shape. Spiral bacteria have a twisted shape, and make up one of the three general groups of bacteria categorized by their cellular shape.

28. B: Clostridium perfringens. Clostridium perfringens is a bacterium that is called tissue gas when it is present in a corpse (postmortem). This bacterium is easily transmitted from one body to another if the trocar is not disinfected between uses. The bacterium Streptococcus pyogenes can be transmitted from large respiratory droplets, and infected persons can develop streptococcal sore throat or rheumatic fever. Clostridium tetani is a bacterium transmitted by spores that can enter the body through needle sticks and puncture wounds. It is also called tetanus (lockjaw). Staphylococcus aureus is the bacterium present in skin abscesses, furuncles, and carbuncles, and can be transmitted by infiltrating lesions in the skin and mucous membranes.

29. B: Morphology. Morphology is the study of the material character (size, shape, and form) of a life form. Mycology is the study of fungi, molds, and yeast. Virology is the study of the tiniest of all non-cellular living organisms known as viruses. Immunology is the study of the resistance or susceptibility of a human or animal to disease.

30. D: Cold. The use of reduced temperatures, including the use of freezers, will not destroy bacteria; cold is not bactericidal. It has only been demonstrated to be bacteriostatic; it merely slows the growth of bacteria. Dry heat involves the use of a hot air oven. It is more effective at destroying bacteria than cold. Moist heat is more bactericidal than dry heat or cold, and it is faster than both of them. An autoclave uses steam under pressure, and is the most bactericidal of the physical methods listed.

31. C: Droplet. The spread of infection through the creation of a droplet in a host and the movement of the droplet to another host is a form of direct transmission. Direct transmission occurs when the life form causing the disease is outside the host for a short period of time and is directly transmitted from one host to another. Food can transmit a microorganism when it is eaten by the host, and this form of transmission of infection is indirect since the organism causing the disease is indirectly passed from one host to another. Fomites are inorganic objects such as forks, countertops, door knobs, etc. that may have microorganisms left by a host on them. These microorganisms can be indirectly passed to another host. Milk can have bacteria microorganisms in it that can move to another host when the milk is ingested. This is a form of indirect transmission.

32. B: Passive hyperemia. Passive hyperemia is a condition that occurs when a malady causes excess blood to stay in a body part, preventing normal drainage. Thrombosis is the condition of reduced blood passage due to a blood clot (thrombus) inside a blood vessel. Active hyperemia is the condition when surplus blood is purposefully taken by blood vessels to an area such as a muscle during exercise. It is not the result of a disease. An embolism is a condition that occurs when a thrombus causes a stoppage in the flow in a blood vessel by blocking the passageway.

33. D: Hemothorax. A hemothorax is when blood pools in the pleural cavity of a human being, typically as a result of an injury. Epistaxis is a bloody nose that occurs when blood pools in the nasal region. Hemopericardium is the condition in which blood pools in the pericardial sac of the heart muscle, and is often seen in an autopsy. Hemoperitoneum is the condition that occurs when blood collects in a person's peritoneal cavity.

34. A: Endogenous. When hemolysis of red blood cells occurs in a corpse and the result is post-mortem stain, the coloring matter pigment made from inside the body is referred to as endogenous. Fomites are non-living objects such as forks, countertops, door knobs, etc. They may have microorganisms on them left by a host that can be indirectly passed to another host. Atrophy is the condition that is characterized by a reduction in size or shrinking of a muscle or a part of the body. Exogenous pigments are those that originate from outside the location they infiltrate.

35. B: Vesicle. A vesicle is a diminutive lesion of raised skin with fluid inside of it, such as a blister. A furuncle is an infection deep in the skin, such as an abscess or boil. An ulcer is a necrosis confined to a small area on the skin or on a mucous membrane. A carbuncle is two or more adjacent furuncles located in the deeper layers of the skin.

36. D: Leucopenia. Leucopenia is a condition in which a person has a diminished white blood cell count, so there is a decrease in the number of infection-fighting cells (leukocytes) in the blood. Hemophilia is a condition characterized by the failure of one's blood to clot appropriately. Leukemia is a form of cancer in which uncharacteristically high numbers of white blood cells are produced in undeveloped forms, meaning the blood and/or bone marrow are not functioning properly. Polycythemia is a condition characterized by an atypical amplification of the number of red blood cells or total red blood cell volume.

37. D: Hepatitis B. Hepatitis B is a viral ailment that affects the functionality of the liver, and is generally more severe than Hepatitis A. Hepatitis B is directly transmitted from host to host through infected body fluids such as saliva, blood, or semen that enter through broken skin. Hemophilia is a disease that results in a bleeding disorder characterized by the inability of one's blood to clot properly. Hepatitis A is a viral disease affecting the liver that is spread principally through food or water. A hemorrhage is a condition characterized by profuse, uncontrollable blood loss from the blood vessels.

38. A: Encephalitis. Encephalitis is a neurotropic viral disease that affects the cranial cavity by causing an engorgement and swelling of the brain tissue. Meningitis is a bacterial or viral ailment that results in an irritation of the protective membranes encasing the brain and spine (meninges). Myelitis is a disease characterized by irritation of the spine, which negatively impacts the functionality of the central nervous system. Poliomyelitis (polio) is a viral malady that impacts the function of nerve tissue and can lead to limited or complete paralysis.

39. C: Skin. The integumentary system is the organ that includes the skin, hair, nails, sweat glands, and sebaceous glands. It encases the entire body of the organism and has sensory and protective functions. The pleural cavity is comprised of the sectional, defined limits of empty space that surround the lungs. The heart is a well-developed organ that is mainly composed of muscle tissue, and it is a fundamental part of the cardiovascular circulatory system. The epididymis is a tubular component of the male reproductive duct structure that serves as a passageway and storage site for sperm.

40. C: Diffusion. Diffusion refers to the movement of molecules from a region of high measurable concentration to a different locale with low measurable concentration. Hydrolysis is a chemical change that occurs as a result of the introduction of water. Cell walls burst and their water is released. It is a very significant component of tissue decomposition. Saturation is an explanatory term used to describe a solution that has absorbed all the solvent it can. A compound is matter that contains two or more components that are chemically integrated.

41. A: Saturation. Saturation is an explanatory term used to describe a solution that has absorbed all the solvent it can. Sublimation is the direct conversion of a solid to a gas or a gas to a solid. The matter does not go through the liquid phase. Inflammation describes the condition of a living body that has stimulated itself into a state of resistance in which engorgement and calor become noticeable physical characteristics. Binary fission is the means by which most bacteria reproduce.

42. D: Hydrolysis. Hydrolysis is a chemical change that occurs as a result of the introduction of water. Cell walls burst and their water is released. It is a very significant component of tissue decomposition. Vaporization is the term used to describe the transition of liquid matter to gaseous matter. Diffusion refers to the movement of molecules from a region of high measurable concentration to a region of low measurable concentration. Adsorption is the bonding of molecules from a gas or liquid. It is accomplished by passing the molecules over the outer layer of a surface and using filtration to capture the intended molecules.

43. A: Aldehydes, alcohols, and phenols. The four major types of preservatives used in embalming fluids are formaldehyde, aldehydes, alcohols, and phenols. Sterols are macrobiotic molecules that are present in plants and animals; they are not a preservative used in embalming fluid. Lipids are organic compounds present in plants and animals that are insoluble in water. They are an important part of cell membranes, but are not used as preservatives in embalming fluid.

44. B: 37; 40. The 100 percent formalin mixture used in embalming is 37 percent HCHO gas by weight and 40 percent HCHO gas by volume.

45. D: Both A: and C:. Phalanges is the term used to refer to the complexly integrated system of various bones that shape the fingers and toes. The phalanges of the foot are the assorted bones that make up the toes and the phalanges of the hand are the bones that constitute the fingers. The location of the elbow on the arm is medial, not distal, and it doesn't include any phalanges. Instead,

it is a descriptive term for the section of the arm connecting three bones: the ulna and the radius from below and the humerus from above.

46. B: Pelvic girdle. The pelvic girdle is an assembly of bones collectively referred to as the hip that are arranged to attach the trunk and legs, and includes a pair of coxal bones called the os coxa. The patella (knee cap) is a bulky sesamoid bone to which tendons are attached. It allows for joint extension of the leg. The phalanges of the foot are the assorted bones that make up the toes and the phalanges of the hand are the bones that constitute the fingers. The circle of Willis is a pattern of arterial configuration found in the lower region of the base of the brain.

47. A: Not moveable. Synarthroses are skeletal links that are not moveable, are unbending, and are held together by unyielding connective tissue. Amphiarthroses are skeletal links that are somewhat moveable. They are held together by connective tissue that allows some articulation. Diarthroses are skeletal links that are very moveable, allowing for a full range of articulation in a joint.

48. A: Median plane. The median plane partitions the body perpendicularly in proportioned segments on both the left and right side. A coronal plane (frontal plane) is any perpendicular plane that separates the body into ventral and dorsal segments. The transverse plane (horizontal plane) partitions the body into superior and inferior segments.

49. C: Pathological anatomy. Pathological anatomy is the division of anatomical studies that focuses on how a disease brings forth various structural changes to the body as it progresses. Regional anatomy involves studying a particular area of the body by sub-dividing it into components or partitions that relate to each other. Gross anatomy is the division of anatomical science that studies the components of the body on a macroscopic level without the help of any visual aid instrument. Systemic anatomy is the division of anatomical science that observes the different systems of the body—such as the organ systems or the cardiovascular system—and concentrates on providing a broad overview of the system as part of the complete body.

50. A: Hormones. The endocrine system manufactures hormones from different glands that are transported all over the body and direct chemical communication in the body. Red blood cells are formed in the bone marrow. White blood cells are created in the bone marrow. Bile is a solution formed by the liver that accumulates in the gall bladder and is discharged into the small intestine through the bile ducts.

51. C: The femoral artery is commonly used as a main injection site in embalming. Although the iliac, ulnar, and aortic arteries are sometimes used, this is uncommon. They are not the main arteries used in embalming.

52. B: Because of the heat it emits, an electric spatula can cause burns unless you use it carefully and liberally apply massage cream to the skin before use.

53. B: The correct formula is to multiply 128 (the ounces per gallon) by the solution percentage (2 percent) and divide that value by the index of the fluid.

54. D: Intermittent drainage will provide better distribution of the fluid, increase saturation in the tissues, and help with the removal of clots. It will not affect the organs enough to make aspiration unnecessary.

55. C: The left and right jugular are veins. They are not used for injection, but for drainage.

56. A: The first thing that needs to be done is to remove the cotton or other absorbent material left in the eye socket by the tissue bank enucleator. This is usually only temporarily absorbent, and has typically spilled out by the time the body is being prepared.

57. C: The stomach is one of the four organs accessed using trocar guides during the aspiration process.

58. D: All of the choices are inexpert tests for death when the equipment needed for expert tests is not present. An inexpert test not listed is feeling for a pulse.

59. A: Closing the mouth and eyes is a necessary step to help give the deceased a natural appearance. None of the other treatments can be done if permission to embalm the deceased has been denied.

60. C: The same arterial embalming fluids are used to embalm babies and adults. A needle injector can't be used on a baby as the bones are too soft; positioning both hands over the body would not be a natural pose for a baby; and the ascending aorta is not an injection site on an adult.

61. A: Sometimes, a partial autopsy is done on only the thorax and not the abdomen. There are no autopsies done on appendages, and the neck is usually part of an autopsy of the torso.

62. C: Pre-injection and co-injection are not categories of embalming, but are part of the arterial embalming process. Autopsy embalming is not an embalming category.

63. D: Humectants are the only type of fluid listed that help prevent dehydration and retain tissue moisture.

64. D: Hypodermic injection is used in any tissue that does not show signs of preservation. These tissues may include the torso walls in an autopsied body.

65. A: Physiognomy is the correct answer. Physiology is the study of living systems. Restorative art is the practice of restoring something to its original state. Facial positioning is a fictional term.

66. B: The eyelids meet two-thirds of the way down the eye, but do not overlap. The top lids are not pulled all the way down as is commonly believed.

67. B: If the tissue is not firm and dry, there is no base on which to do the reconstructive work. When sutures will be done and any necessary wax or other restorative substances will be used, a firm and dry base allows these substances to be applied easily and also to retain their shape. This allows them to better perform their purpose.

68. A: Dimples are a natural marking on the face. The other choices are all considered acquired facial markings, as they typically appear with age.

69. D: Horizontal is not a facial profile. A vertical profile is a balanced profile in which the forehead, upper lip, and chin align on an imaginary line. A convex profile is one in which the forehead and chin recede from a prominent upper lip. A concave profile is one in which the forehead and chin protrude farther than the upper lip.

70. D: All of the choices are good reasons to take the time to do the restorative work necessary to create an appropriate way for people to see the deceased, which will help them with their grief.

71. B: When a family wants to see the deceased before you have time to do an extensive hair restoration, using a scarf on a woman or a head bandage on a man is an acceptable way to present the deceased. These familiar articles are items that cover injuries or abnormalities. People can relate to a scarf or a bandage more than an inadequate attempt at restoration.

72. C: The complimentary color to red on the color wheel is green. Although the most common color for concealer is beige, complimentary colors work best on discolored areas. Once these areas have been neutralized in this manner, they can then be covered with a natural color of makeup.

73. C: A stipple brush, with its stiff and slightly separated tips, will provide an appearance similar to pores in the skin. A tapered, flat tip, or pointed brush will not provide this effect.

74. A: The width of the base of the nose equals the width of the eye. The eye is one half the width of the mouth, one fifth the width of the face, and equal to the distance between the eyes.

75. D: The basket weave stitch has a crisscross design that provides the best base for restorative wax. A worm stitch and a purse string stitch are used to close a wound, and a temporary stitch would not serve as a base if it was removed.

76. B: The points of entry and exit form the letter "X," and this pattern of stitches can help reduce swelling in the neck.

77. C. Massage cream thinned with a little mineral oil will work well to fill in tissue subcutaneously. Water will not fill in tissue, and will probably make it worse. Wax is too thick to inject hypodermically, and tissue filler solvent will not fill in tissue.

78. D: When there is extensive damage to the face and restoration is not possible, all of the actions listed are good alternatives to give family members the peace of knowing for sure that it is indeed their family member.

79. A: Although syphilis can be contracted through kissing, placental transmission, and blood transfusions, approximately 95 percent of cases are due to sexual intercourse involving direct contact with the fluids or lesions of an infected individual.

80. C: Although all of the choices are bodily fluids, the only one listed on the CDC's list of hazardous fluids is spinal fluid.

81. A: OSHA (Occupational Safety and Health Administration) is the agency that oversees safety in the workplace. This includes developing standards to prevent the transmission of communicable diseases. The CDC is the Centers for Disease Control. The NRA establishes guidelines for the safe handling of firearms but has nothing to do with preventing the spread of disease. The ADA is the American Disabilities Act, which sets guidelines for making facilities accessible to those with disabilities or handicaps.

82. A: Hepatitis A is classified as highly contagious, hepatitis B and C are mildly contagious, and there is no such thing as hepatitis D.

83. B: Bleach is the best disinfectant for many organisms, including those present in HIV.

84. D: Kaposi's sarcoma is most often seen in those with AIDS. Though the reason for the correlation is unclear, it may be because of the breakdown of the immune system.

85. C: The three parts of healthy human cells are the nucleus, cytoplasm, and a cell (plasma) membrane. DNA and RNA are part of the nucleus, and protoplasm is comprised of both nucleoplasm and cytoplasm.

86. A: AIDS cannot be transmitted through the saliva of an infected person. Sexual contact and contact with an infected person's blood can transmit the disease to another person. A pregnant woman with AIDS can also transmit the virus to her unborn child through the placenta.

87. B: Edema is defined as excess fluid in those spaces. Plasma is a fluid contained in the blood. A hernia is not an excess of fluid but a protrusion of tissue, and sepsis is poisoning of the blood.

88. B: The respiratory system is most affected by influenza, and typically results in nasal and breathing problems. The respiratory system is susceptible because it is an open-ended system that comes into contact with the environment.

89. D: At this time, only corneal transplants, dura mater, and human growth hormone from a contaminated donor are known to be modes of transmission for Creutzfeldt-Jakob disease.

90. C: Cardiovascular diseases are the most common causes of death in the U.S. and other industrialized nations.

91. A: The lungs are part of the respiratory system.

92. A: The chemical composition of embalming fluids makes the vapors heavy. Therefore, the best place for an exhaust fan is close to the embalming table near the floor. Many embalming rooms have a fan not only there but also near or in the ceiling, but if you have only one, it should be near the floor and close to the embalming table.

93. B: Autopsy gels have the same chemical composition as cavity fluid but are in a gel form to make applying the gels to the autopsied surfaces of the body and viscera easier.

94. C: Pre-injection and co-injection fluids also work well with arterial preservative fluids, but cavity fluids have higher concentrations of preservatives and disinfectants.

95. D: Humectants are not arterial fluid preservatives but modifying agents, which work with arterial fluids to help offset dehydration.

96. B: Although the circle of Willis is exposed, it is the name of a formation of arteries and is not an opening. The foramen magnum is the large opening exposed at the base of the skull, where it meets the spinal cord.

97. B: The heart is the center of the circulatory system. The lungs are central to the respiratory system. Although arteries and veins are part of the circulatory system, they cannot operate without the heart.

98. A: They are located under the sternocleidomastoid muscle. The trachea is deeper and centered in the body; it is not located to the left or right of the center line of the body. The sternum is also in the center of the body, and is lower than the carotid and jugular vessels. The ulnar artery is in the lower arm.

99. C: The right and left iliac are exposed and easily accessible for embalming the lower extremities. As such, it's not necessary to use the femoral vessels. The ulnar arteries are usually not injected since they are in the wrist, and embalming of the arms is achieved through the axillary, brachial, or subclavian arteries. The jugular vessels are veins and are not injected; their arterial counterparts are the right and left carotids.

100. D: Capillaries are the third type of blood vessels. The atria and ventricles are part of the heart but are not blood vessels. Valves are found in the heart and the veins, but are not vessels themselves.

Secret Key #1 - Time is Your Greatest Enemy

Pace Yourself

Wear a watch. At the beginning of the test, check the time (or start a chronometer on your watch to count the minutes), and check the time after every few questions to make sure you are "on schedule."

If you are forced to speed up, do it efficiently. Usually one or more answer choices can be eliminated without too much difficulty. Above all, don't panic. Don't speed up and just begin guessing at random choices. By pacing yourself, and continually monitoring your progress against your watch, you will always know exactly how far ahead or behind you are with your available time. If you find that you are one minute behind on the test, don't skip one question without spending any time on it, just to catch back up. Take 15 fewer seconds on the next four questions, and after four questions you'll have caught back up. Once you catch back up, you can continue working each problem at your normal pace.

Furthermore, don't dwell on the problems that you were rushed on. If a problem was taking up too much time and you made a hurried guess, it must be difficult. The difficult questions are the ones you are most likely to miss anyway, so it isn't a big loss. It is better to end with more time than you need than to run out of time.

Lastly, sometimes it is beneficial to slow down if you are constantly getting ahead of time. You are always more likely to catch a careless mistake by working more slowly than quickly, and among very high-scoring test takers (those who are likely to have lots of time left over), careless errors affect the score more than mastery of material.

Secret Key #2 - Guessing is not Guesswork

You probably know that guessing is a good idea - unlike other standardized tests, there is no penalty for getting a wrong answer. Even if you have no idea about a question, you still have a 20-25% chance of getting it right.

Most test takers do not understand the impact that proper guessing can have on their score. Unless you score extremely high, guessing will significantly contribute to your final score.

Monkeys Take the Test

What most test takers don't realize is that to insure that 20-25% chance, you have to guess randomly. If you put 20 monkeys in a room to take this test, assuming they answered once per question and behaved themselves, on average they would get 20-25% of the questions correct. Put 20 test takers in the room, and the average will be much lower among guessed questions. Why?

1. The test writers intentionally writes deceptive answer choices that "look" right. A test taker has no idea about a question, so picks the "best looking" answer, which is often wrong. The monkey has no idea what looks good and what doesn't, so will consistently be lucky about 20-25% of the time.
2. Test takers will eliminate answer choices from the guessing pool based on a hunch or intuition. Simple but correct answers often get excluded, leaving a 0% chance of being correct. The monkey has no clue, and often gets lucky with the best choice.

This is why the process of elimination endorsed by most test courses is flawed and detrimental to your performance- test takers don't guess, they make an ignorant stab in the dark that is usually worse than random.

$5 Challenge

Let me introduce one of the most valuable ideas of this course- the $5 challenge:

You only mark your "best guess" if you are willing to bet $5 on it.
You only eliminate choices from guessing if you are willing to bet $5 on it.

Why $5? Five dollars is an amount of money that is small yet not insignificant, and can really add up fast (20 questions could cost you $100). Likewise, each answer choice on one question of the test will have a small impact on your overall score, but it can really add up to a lot of points in the end.

The process of elimination IS valuable. The following shows your chance of guessing it right:

If you eliminate wrong answer choices until only this many remain:	1	2	3
Chance of getting it correct:	100%	50%	33%

However, if you accidentally eliminate the right answer or go on a hunch for an incorrect answer, your chances drop dramatically: to 0%. By guessing among all the answer choices, you are GUARANTEED to have a shot at the right answer.

That's why the $5 test is so valuable- if you give up the advantage and safety of a pure guess, it had better be worth the risk.

What we still haven't covered is how to be sure that whatever guess you make is truly random. Here's the easiest way:

Always pick the first answer choice among those remaining.

Such a technique means that you have decided, **before you see a single test question**, exactly how you are going to guess- and since the order of choices tells you nothing about which one is correct, this guessing technique is perfectly random.

This section is not meant to scare you away from making educated guesses or eliminating choices- you just need to define when a choice is worth eliminating. The $5 test, along with a pre-defined random guessing strategy, is the best way to make sure you reap all of the benefits of guessing.

Secret Key #3 - Practice Smarter, Not Harder

Many test takers delay the test preparation process because they dread the awful amounts of practice time they think necessary to succeed on the test. We have refined an effective method that will take you only a fraction of the time.

There are a number of "obstacles" in your way to succeed. Among these are answering questions, finishing in time, and mastering test-taking strategies. All must be executed on the day of the test at peak performance, or your score will suffer. The test is a mental marathon that has a large impact on your future.

Just like a marathon runner, it is important to work your way up to the full challenge. So first you just worry about questions, and then time, and finally strategy:

Success Strategy

1. Find a good source for practice tests.
2. If you are willing to make a larger time investment, consider using more than one study guide- often the different approaches of multiple authors will help you "get" difficult concepts.
3. Take a practice test with no time constraints, with all study helps "open book." Take your time with questions and focus on applying strategies.
4. Take a practice test with time constraints, with all guides "open book."
5. Take a final practice test with no open material and time limits

If you have time to take more practice tests, just repeat step 5. By gradually exposing yourself to the full rigors of the test environment, you will condition your mind to the stress of test day and maximize your success.

Secret Key #4 - Prepare, Don't Procrastinate

Let me state an obvious fact: if you take the test three times, you will get three different scores. This is due to the way you feel on test day, the level of preparedness you have, and, despite the test writers' claims to the contrary, some tests WILL be easier for you than others.

Since your future depends so much on your score, you should maximize your chances of success. In order to maximize the likelihood of success, you've got to prepare in advance. This means taking practice tests and spending time learning the information and test taking strategies you will need to succeed.

Never take the test as a "practice" test, expecting that you can just take it again if you need to. Feel free to take sample tests on your own, but when you go to take the official test, be prepared, be focused, and do your best the first time!

Secret Key #5 - Test Yourself

Everyone knows that time is money. There is no need to spend too much of your time or too little of your time preparing for the test. You should only spend as much of your precious time preparing as is necessary for you to get the score you need.

Once you have taken a practice test under real conditions of time constraints, then you will know if you are ready for the test or not.

If you have scored extremely high the first time that you take the practice test, then there is not much point in spending countless hours studying. You are already there.

Benchmark your abilities by retaking practice tests and seeing how much you have improved. Once you score high enough to guarantee success, then you are ready.

If you have scored well below where you need, then knuckle down and begin studying in earnest. Check your improvement regularly through the use of practice tests under real conditions. Above all, don't worry, panic, or give up. The key is perseverance!

Then, when you go to take the test, remain confident and remember how well you did on the practice tests. If you can score high enough on a practice test, then you can do the same on the real thing.

General Strategies

The most important thing you can do is to ignore your fears and jump into the test immediately- do not be overwhelmed by any strange-sounding terms. You have to jump into the test like jumping into a pool- all at once is the easiest way.

Make Predictions

As you read and understand the question, try to guess what the answer will be. Remember that several of the answer choices are wrong, and once you begin reading them, your mind will immediately become cluttered with answer choices designed to throw you off. Your mind is typically the most focused immediately after you have read the question and digested its contents. If you can, try to predict what the correct answer will be. You may be surprised at what you can predict.

Quickly scan the choices and see if your prediction is in the listed answer choices. If it is, then you can be quite confident that you have the right answer. It still won't hurt to check the other answer choices, but most of the time, you've got it!

Answer the Question

It may seem obvious to only pick answer choices that answer the question, but the test writers can create some excellent answer choices that are wrong. Don't pick an answer just because it sounds right, or you believe it to be true. It MUST answer the question. Once you've made your selection, always go back and check it against the question and make sure that you didn't misread the question, and the answer choice does answer the question posed.

Benchmark

After you read the first answer choice, decide if you think it sounds correct or not. If it doesn't, move on to the next answer choice. If it does, mentally mark that answer choice. This doesn't mean that you've definitely selected it as your answer choice, it just means that it's the best you've seen thus far. Go ahead and read the next choice. If the next choice is worse than the one you've already selected, keep going to the next answer choice. If the next choice is better than the choice you've already selected, mentally mark the new answer choice as your best guess.

The first answer choice that you select becomes your standard. Every other answer choice must be benchmarked against that standard. That choice is correct until proven otherwise by another answer choice beating it out. Once you've decided that no other answer choice seems as good, do one final check to ensure that your answer choice answers the question posed.

Valid Information

Don't discount any of the information provided in the question. Every piece of information may be necessary to determine the correct answer. None of the information in the question is there to throw you off (while the answer choices will certainly have information to throw you off). If two seemingly unrelated topics are discussed, don't ignore either. You can be confident there is a relationship, or it wouldn't be included in the question, and you are probably going to have to determine what is that relationship to find the answer.

Avoid "Fact Traps"

Don't get distracted by a choice that is factually true. Your search is for the answer that answers the question. Stay focused and don't fall for an answer that is true but incorrect. Always go back to the question and make sure you're choosing an answer that actually answers the question and is not just a true statement. An answer can be factually correct, but it MUST answer the question asked. Additionally, two answers can both be seemingly correct, so be sure to read all of the answer choices, and make sure that you get the one that BEST answers the question.

Milk the Question
Some of the questions may throw you completely off. They might deal with a subject you have not been exposed to, or one that you haven't reviewed in years. While your lack of knowledge about the subject will be a hindrance, the question itself can give you many clues that will help you find the correct answer. Read the question carefully and look for clues. Watch particularly for adjectives and nouns describing difficult terms or words that you don't recognize. Regardless of if you completely understand a word or not, replacing it with a synonym either provided or one you more familiar with may help you to understand what the questions are asking. Rather than wracking your mind about specific detailed information concerning a difficult term or word, try to use mental substitutes that are easier to understand.

The Trap of Familiarity
Don't just choose a word because you recognize it. On difficult questions, you may not recognize a number of words in the answer choices. The test writers don't put "make-believe" words on the test; so don't think that just because you only recognize all the words in one answer choice means that answer choice must be correct. If you only recognize words in one answer choice, then focus on that one. Is it correct? Try your best to determine if it is correct. If it is, that is great, but if it doesn't, eliminate it. Each word and answer choice you eliminate increases your chances of getting the question correct, even if you then have to guess among the unfamiliar choices.

Eliminate Answers
Eliminate choices as soon as you realize they are wrong. But be careful! Make sure you consider all of the possible answer choices. Just because one appears right, doesn't mean that the next one won't be even better! The test writers will usually put more than one good answer choice for every question, so read all of them. Don't worry if you are stuck between two that seem right. By getting down to just two remaining possible choices, your odds are now 50/50. Rather than wasting too much time, play the odds. You are guessing, but guessing wisely, because you've been able to knock out some of the answer choices that you know are wrong. If you are eliminating choices and realize that the last answer choice you are left with is also obviously wrong, don't panic. Start over and consider each choice again. There may easily be something that you missed the first time and will realize on the second pass.

Tough Questions
If you are stumped on a problem or it appears too hard or too difficult, don't waste time. Move on! Remember though, if you can quickly check for obviously incorrect answer choices, your chances of guessing correctly are greatly improved. Before you completely give up, at least try to knock out a couple of possible answers. Eliminate what you can and then guess at the remaining answer choices before moving on.

Brainstorm
If you get stuck on a difficult question, spend a few seconds quickly brainstorming. Run through the complete list of possible answer choices. Look at each choice and ask yourself, "Could this answer the question satisfactorily?" Go through each answer choice and consider it independently of the other. By systematically going through all possibilities, you may find something that you would otherwise overlook. Remember that when you get stuck, it's important to try to keep moving.

Read Carefully

Understand the problem. Read the question and answer choices carefully. Don't miss the question because you misread the terms. You have plenty of time to read each question thoroughly and make sure you understand what is being asked. Yet a happy medium must be attained, so don't waste too much time. You must read carefully, but efficiently.

Face Value

When in doubt, use common sense. Always accept the situation in the problem at face value. Don't read too much into it. These problems will not require you to make huge leaps of logic. The test writers aren't trying to throw you off with a cheap trick. If you have to go beyond creativity and make a leap of logic in order to have an answer choice answer the question, then you should look at the other answer choices. Don't overcomplicate the problem by creating theoretical relationships or explanations that will warp time or space. These are normal problems rooted in reality. It's just that the applicable relationship or explanation may not be readily apparent and you have to figure things out. Use your common sense to interpret anything that isn't clear.

Prefixes

If you're having trouble with a word in the question or answer choices, try dissecting it. Take advantage of every clue that the word might include. Prefixes and suffixes can be a huge help. Usually they allow you to determine a basic meaning. Pre- means before, post- means after, pro - is positive, de- is negative. From these prefixes and suffixes, you can get an idea of the general meaning of the word and try to put it into context. Beware though of any traps. Just because con is the opposite of pro, doesn't necessarily mean congress is the opposite of progress!

Hedge Phrases

Watch out for critical "hedge" phrases, such as likely, may, can, will often, sometimes, often, almost, mostly, usually, generally, rarely, sometimes. Question writers insert these hedge phrases to cover every possibility. Often an answer choice will be wrong simply because it leaves no room for exception. Avoid answer choices that have definitive words like "exactly," and "always".

Switchback Words

Stay alert for "switchbacks". These are the words and phrases frequently used to alert you to shifts in thought. The most common switchback word is "but". Others include although, however, nevertheless, on the other hand, even though, while, in spite of, despite, regardless of.

New Information

Correct answer choices will rarely have completely new information included. Answer choices typically are straightforward reflections of the material asked about and will directly relate to the question. If a new piece of information is included in an answer choice that doesn't even seem to relate to the topic being asked about, then that answer choice is likely incorrect. All of the information needed to answer the question is usually provided for you, and so you should not have to make guesses that are unsupported or choose answer choices that require unknown information that cannot be reasoned on its own.

Time Management

On technical questions, don't get lost on the technical terms. Don't spend too much time on any one question. If you don't know what a term means, then since you don't have a dictionary, odds are you aren't going to get much further. You should immediately recognize terms as whether or not you know them. If you don't, work with the other clues that you have, the other answer choices and terms provided, but don't waste too much time trying to figure out a difficult term.

Contextual Clues
Look for contextual clues. An answer can be right but not correct. The contextual clues will help you find the answer that is most right and is correct. Understand the context in which a phrase or statement is made. This will help you make important distinctions.

Don't Panic
Panicking will not answer any questions for you. Therefore, it isn't helpful. When you first see the question, if your mind goes blank, take a deep breath. Force yourself to mechanically go through the steps of solving the problem and using the strategies you've learned.

Pace Yourself
Don't get clock fever. It's easy to be overwhelmed when you're looking at a page full of questions, your mind is full of random thoughts and feeling confused, and the clock is ticking down faster than you would like. Calm down and maintain the pace that you have set for yourself. As long as you are on track by monitoring your pace, you are guaranteed to have enough time for yourself. When you get to the last few minutes of the test, it may seem like you won't have enough time left, but if you only have as many questions as you should have left at that point, then you're right on track!

Answer Selection
The best way to pick an answer choice is to eliminate all of those that are wrong, until only one is left and confirm that is the correct answer. Sometimes though, an answer choice may immediately look right. Be careful! Take a second to make sure that the other choices are not equally obvious. Don't make a hasty mistake. There are only two times that you should stop before checking other answers. First is when you are positive that the answer choice you have selected is correct. Second is when time is almost out and you have to make a quick guess!

Check Your Work
Since you will probably not know every term listed and the answer to every question, it is important that you get credit for the ones that you do know. Don't miss any questions through careless mistakes. If at all possible, try to take a second to look back over your answer selection and make sure you've selected the correct answer choice and haven't made a costly careless mistake (such as marking an answer choice that you didn't mean to mark). This quick double check should more than pay for itself in caught mistakes for the time it costs.

Beware of Directly Quoted Answers
Sometimes an answer choice will repeat word for word a portion of the question or reference section. However, beware of such exact duplication – it may be a trap! More than likely, the correct choice will paraphrase or summarize a point, rather than being exactly the same wording.

Slang
Scientific sounding answers are better than slang ones. An answer choice that begins "To compare the outcomes..." is much more likely to be correct than one that begins "Because some people insisted..."

Extreme Statements
Avoid wild answers that throw out highly controversial ideas that are proclaimed as established fact. An answer choice that states the "process should be used in certain situations, if..." is much

more likely to be correct than one that states the "process should be discontinued completely." The first is a calm rational statement and doesn't even make a definitive, uncompromising stance, using a hedge word "if" to provide wiggle room, whereas the second choice is a radical idea and far more extreme.

Answer Choice Families

When you have two or more answer choices that are direct opposites or parallels, one of them is usually the correct answer. For instance, if one answer choice states "x increases" and another answer choice states "x decreases" or "y increases," then those two or three answer choices are very similar in construction and fall into the same family of answer choices. A family of answer choices is when two or three answer choices are very similar in construction, and yet often have a directly opposite meaning. Usually the correct answer choice will be in that family of answer choices. The "odd man out" or answer choice that doesn't seem to fit the parallel construction of the other answer choices is more likely to be incorrect.

Special Report: Additional Bonus Material

Due to our efforts to try to keep this book to a manageable length, we've created a link that will give you access to all of your additional bonus material.

Please visit http://www.mometrix.com/bonus948/funeral to access the information.